Contents

Nursing Research

A skills-based introduction

COLLETTE CLIFFORD
Senior Nurse Education Manager

STEPHEN GOUGH
Librarian

Queen Elizabeth School of Nursing, Birmingham

Prentice Hall

New York London Toronto Sydney Tokyo Singapore

First published 1990 by
Prentice Hall International (UK) Ltd,
66 Wood Lane End, Hemel Hempstead,
Hertfordshire, HP2 4RG
A division of
Simon & Schuster International Group

Typeset by Inforum Typesetting, Portsmouth
Printed and bound in Great Britain by
BPCC Wheatons Ltd, Exeter

1733439

British Library Cataloguing in Publication Data

Clifford, Collette
    Nursing research.
    1. Medicine. Nursing. Research
    I. Title   II. Gough, Stephen
    610.73072

    ISBN 0–13–629114–7

1 2 3 4 5 94 93 92 91 90

Acknowledgements

This book is dedicated to the students of the Queen Elizabeth School of Nursing and the staff of the Central Birmingham Health Authority who, by their constant questioning and search for advice when undertaking research studies, identified the need for a book of this nature.

Thanks are extended to those people who gave time and energy in reviewing draft copies of the book. Kate Fotheringham and Mavis Hartley gave useful comments and advice. The technical advice from Caroline Hicks was most beneficial and reassuring at a time when the end product seemed far from complete. In addition Lynn Copcutt and Jenny Clark gave crucial support in the initial stages.

Finally, grateful thanks are extended to colleagues, friends and families who have given support and encouragement during the preparation of this manuscript.

Introduction

The overall content of this book is based on several years of experience of introducing nursing staff and student nurses to research. The framework is one that has been used with some success in motivating interest in research at an introductory level. The emphasis given to each issue identified in the book reflects areas of uncertainty that have caused particular difficulties for nurses approaching research studies for the first time.

The first chapter gives a general introduction to the topic. In focusing on the 'what, why and who' in nursing research it is hoped that newcomers to the subject may gain insight into the wider issues involved in developing research skills in nursing. The second chapter focuses on research awareness. This is seen to be an important inclusion in an introductory text for study of nursing research that does not necessarily mean undertaking a research project. The aim of a course of study in research may be to enhance awareness of research in general.

The next three chapters focus on the research process. Chapter 3 concentrates on generating research ideas. Nurses approaching research studies for the first time often have more difficulty with this than with any other aspect of the research process. This is followed by a chapter on some of the general practical issues involved in planning research.

Chapter 5 outlines the research process and offers a source of reference for the process as a whole. The outline in this chapter could also be useful for nurses who are learning to read research literature critically, for it offers a framework by which research reports can be analysed.

The chapter on literature searching is the only chapter not written exclusively for newcomers. The comprehensive explanation of how to search literature and the resources available to help nurses in this provides a useful source of reference for anyone involved in research studies.

In examining approaches to research and the methods and techniques deployed in data collection Chapter 7 gives quite a wide range of information. Each of the areas discussed in this chapter could, and do, provide enough material for books in their own right and so the limitations of this chapter are recognised. However, the content reflects the issues that cause concern to nurses approaching research studies at an elementary level and it is not intended for it be a definitive guide on data collection. A short chapter on analysing research data has been included to help nurses understand some of the techniques used by researchers to analyse and present data. This is felt to be important as familiarity with some of the issues identified in Chapter 8 will do much to enhance understanding of research reports using statistical techniques to present data.

Sharing knowledge is a crucial part of research studies. It has been common practice in our school, in common with many others, to place much emphasis on this component as part of research studies. However, it has been our experience that preparation of written material related to research has caused considerable anxiety to those nurses expected to write essays on research, research proposals or research reports. In addition, the presentation of information gained through research studies can, and does, cause extreme anxiety to newcomers to nursing research. Consequently, although a chapter on presentation skills is not common in texts on research we see this as an important inclusion in this book. Both aspects have formed part of programmes of research studies, for the sharing of research knowledge is crucial if we are to enhance the professional knowledge base.

As knowledge of research increases so the need to change practices may be identified. Consequently, in the final chapter, the use of change theory has been included to help those nurses who wish to introduce research-based practices into their own area of work.

Because of the variety of material explored in this book each chapter stands alone as a source of reference. There are areas of overlap as some issues identified in earlier chapters are examined in more depth in later sections. Where this occurs the reader is referred to other relevant sections of the book.

In any introductory text the range and depth of material examined is, of necessity, limited. A list of further reading is given at the end of each chapter as a means of overcoming this problem.

It can be seen that in taking a skills-based approach to an introduction to nursing research the emphasis in this book extends beyond the skills required to undertake research in nursing. Other issues seen as important to nurses in the developing and sharing knowledge of research have been explored. The content of the book reflects specific areas identified as causing anxiety by nurses who are beginning studies of research and consequently it is anticipated that it will be a useful reference text for those in this position.

Within this text, in the interest of uniformity of approach, the female pronoun 'she' is used throughout to refer to the nurse.

1　Research in nursing

The interest in research in nursing has grown rapidly in recent years to the extent that all nurses are now encouraged to ensure that their practices reflect knowledge based on research rather than ritualistic practices. In this chapter three aspects of research are explored. The first section describes nursing research. The next two sections explore the increasing interest in research and who can do research in nursing.

What is nursing research?

As the interest in research in nursing has grown the number of definitions and explorations of the topic has increased. Most definitions of research in nursing follow a similar theme, with the search for knowledge being emphasised as a fundamental reason for undertaking research studies. There is a consensus that this search must follow a logical planned format for it to be classed as a research study. This distinguishes research from other types of projects that may be undertaken for the purpose of enquiry. This is important in nursing, for there are many different formats that may be used when undertaking enquiries. For example, a new nursing student may undertake a project to determine the health education facilities available in their district. At the early stage of a course it would not normally be expected for this student to have an extensive knowledge of methods of data collection. Consequently, the means by which the student collects information will be left very much to her own initiative and so the teacher may expect a variety of approaches to be used.

Further analysis of a number of definitions of research shows similar themes emerging through all of them. The emphasis in each varies but, in general terms, there is some note made of research reflecting a scientific process. The word 'scientific' perhaps serves to make research appear somewhat distant from the practice of nursing. The associations with science may be seen as something more common to those used to working in laboratories, rather than to people working with others in a health care setting. The scientific approach to research indicates a situation in which there is control over the factors that are being studied. By exerting this control, the researcher is attempting to predict what will happen following a planned sequence of events. In using such an approach the researcher is in fact undertaking an experiment.

Although the notion of conducting an experiment is familiar to many of us it does represent quite a complex approach to research. This can easily be illustrated in relation to our own experiences. In a laboratory setting in our school-days we may have performed experiments by mixing a little of substance A with a little of substance B and producing substance C. If this was done on ten occasions and, if each occasion produced the same result, then we would feel fairly confident that on the eleventh occasion the same result would occur. In other words, we would be predicting the outcome based on the findings of our experiment. If using an experimental approach to nursing research the researcher will approach the study in a similarly controlled way. All factors should be monitored closely and the pattern of events analysed to determine the outcome on each occasion. The goal of the research would be to predict the outcome of a given situation based on the findings of the experimental study.

There are very practical implications for this type of research in nursing but, when studying people, it is not so easy to have control over all the variables involved in the experiment in the same way as it is in the laboratory when working with chemical substances. For example, the nurse searching for the perfect technique to enhance healing of the infected wound may choose to carry out an experimental study to determine which is the most effective dressing to use in this situation. She would need to consider a large number of variables including factors such as age, wound site, causative organisms, underlying diseases and so on. The benefits of such research are that a nurse might then be able to predict with some confidence that a particular dressing was the one most likely to promote a quick recovery in her patients with wound infection.

Although studies of this nature have been undertaken there are specific skills demanded of the researcher carrying out experimental studies. Because of the complexity of this there is no long tradition of experimental research in nursing. Consequently, alternative approaches to research, which do not seek to predict outcomes, are more commonly utilised. Rather than attempting to exert control in an experimental situation, for example, the researcher may analyse the relationship between observed events. The term used for this type of study is descriptive research.

Research which analyses relationships between events can be particularly useful in nursing. For example, if there was an outbreak of food poisoning in a unit the infection control nurse might find that two events happened at the same time. That is, the outbreak of food poisoning occurred at the same time that a particular member of staff was on duty. In noting this relationship the nurse has identified factors that can be investigated further. She is not predicting an outbreak of food poisoning each time the member of staff is on duty, she is simply noting an association between the two events. If the nurse wished to identify a link between the outbreak of food poisoning and the personnel responsible for preparing that food she may choose to do so by undertaking an experimental study. It would require the control of an experimental study for the nurse to predict that the food poisoning was directly related to the member of staff on duty.

Descriptive research describes what the researcher observes in a given situation; there is no attempt to manipulate the situation to determine any cause and effect factors. Once information has been gathered it can be analysed in such a way as to determine whether there is a pattern indicating possible relationships between the variables studied.

Whichever approach is taken, the common themes to emerge in any definitions of research is that it is a planned, logical process. Research may be undertaken for the purpose of analysing relationships between events, or for predicting outcomes; it may be seen as a problem-solving process undertaken in the pursuit of knowledge. The 'problem' is the area that is the subject of the study, whether that be the value of a particular wound dressing in an experimental study or, in a descriptive study, the pattern of events in a food poisoning outbreak. In determining the problem area, the researcher would be specific in stating the area of enquiry when planning a study.

Some types of research may not have a clearly defined 'problem' area at the outset. In the pursuit of knowledge the researcher may look for understanding, or meaning, in a given situation. For example, the researcher may observe student nurses during their training programme and closely monitor the students' experience in an attempt to understand what it means to them. This case study approach does not identify a 'problem' area for research; rather, it seeks to add to the body of knowledge by taking an in-depth look at one particular situation.

In summary, research can be seen as a search for knowledge in which the format of the enquiry is logical and clearly defined. A variety of approaches to research can be identified; each should be utilised appropriately in relation to the subject of enquiry.

Why research in nursing? – a historical perspective

An increasing number of nurses are resolving their own uncertainties about research by undertaking research appreciation courses in which their insight and knowledge of the subject can be increased. However, there are still many practising nurses who see research as something new and consequently tend to view it with suspicion. It is recognised that this suspicion may come from uncertainty about what research means, and what the implications of using research are to the nursing profession. Although there is increasing knowledge about the subject among practitioners there remains an element of mystique associated with research in nursing.

The reason for this situation lies in the history of the nursing profession. It is interesting to note that Florence Nightingale is frequently given credit in many research texts for being the first nurse researcher. The statistical work she produced to support her claims for the developing nursing work-force in the early days of organised nursing should be reviewed by any potential recruits to nursing research. It was perhaps unfortunate that in her time Miss Nightingale did not identify the value of encouraging others to take such an analytic approach to their work, concentrating instead upon the practicalities of nursing.

The nurse leaders of the last century were to do much to enhance the establishment of the nursing profession by demonstrating the value of an organised work-force. Despite this there were many other factors that were to impinge on the development of the nursing profession and these can be usefully reviewed to set the subject of nursing research into context.

Conventional nursing histories have given excellent reviews of the origins of organised nursing and in so doing have given many facts relevant to nurses today. In more recent years nurse historians have developed the study of nursing from differing angles, placing the origins of the profession in more general historical, social and political contexts. In taking this stance more insight can be gained into the role of the nurse in society today. This way of reviewing the history of nursing is particularly relevant in relation to the development of research in nursing since the origins of the profession in the latter half of the nineteenth century were very much tied up with the role of women in Victorian society. Consequently, many of the aspects of that society which affected the role of women had a major impact on nursing, which was to become one of the major occupations for women of that day.

The choice of nursing for many reflects attitudes towards caring from times preceding the Victorian era. The origin of the word 'nurse' is simple in that it derives from the verb 'to nourish'; therefore, the caring picture of giving support and comfort fits well with the maternal role. Nursing is commonly viewed as women's work because of this association with the role of the mother in caring and giving comfort which has been the pattern since time immemorial. This is the background against which the role of the nurse in contemporary society has developed. In the latter half of the nineteenth century nursing as a career was eventually accepted by society as a suitable role for women. It has been noted by nurse historians that the emergence of the feminist movement at the same period undoubtedly affected attitudes to the evolving profession. Women could claim, perhaps for the first time, to have a profession of their own. With this claim they had the power to discriminate against men (Abel-Smith, 1960). When the nurse registration act was established in 1919 it left no means available for a man to be admitted to the General Register. It was not until 1937 that the Society of Male Nurses was formed and began a battle for equal status with the female nurse.

The choice of nursing as a career for many of those taking the option in the nineteenth century was not simply to do with individual ability or desire to care. Other factors have been highlighted that may have affected this choice. These include the limited occupational choices at a time of demographic imbalance: there were more women than men in the latter part of the last century and, as this reduced the likelihood of marriage, these women had to find something to do with their lives. Nursing was one option available to them. This stand to create a female profession of nursing might not have been in the best interests of the feminist movement of the day for, as noted by Maggs (1985), the security offered by a female-dominated occupation simply served to reinforce the contemporary belief about women, that their role was limited to one of caring.

This situation in relation to the evolution of the nursing profession offers an explanation as to why research in nursing was relatively slow to develop in this country: nursing was seen as women's work. In the last century it was not the norm for women to go to university; in fact, advanced education for women at that time was certainly not encouraged. Although the wealthier classes actually had a choice, it can be said that domestic pursuits were encouraged while the arts were seen as acceptable pastimes with which to while away the hours. In contrast to this, for example, medical practice was developing as a male mono-poly with a sound educational base. Historians suggest that doctors at that time saw advantages in maintaining the male monopoly, fearing that the entrance of women into the profession would reduce the status of the profession and prob-ably damage existing levels of remuneration. However, it could be that the concept of inequality was beyond the comprehension of many people in Victorian England and so may not have received serious consideration at that time. Nevertheless, subsequent developments in nurse education and the result-ing slow evolution of research as part of everyday practice in nursing can be retraced to these early days of organised nursing.

Over the years attempts to change the status of nurse education have been slowly accepted. There is evidence to suggest that with the development of academic departments in nursing in the UK, education-based nursing research has become established. In historical terms it is hard to pin down the specific beginnings of research in modern nursing. There were no doubt many who had inquiring minds and applied a questioning approach to their work from the outset. This is well illustrated, for example, by Hockey (1985), who indicates how, as a junior nurse, she began to question 'why?', an approach that subsequently led to a high level of expertise in the area of research.

The difficulty in identifying the beginning of formal nursing research activities in this country has been noted by several authors, all of whom stress the relatively short history of research in nursing. Altshul (1984) has outlined research work dating back to the 1950s and in so doing she notes that much of this early research is viewed as seminal by present-day researchers. The Research Discussion Group established by the Royal College of Nursing is seen by Sheahan (1986) as a turning point in formalising support for nurse researchers. From this point on he traces distinctive developments in the 1960s, as research posts were created by key institutions including the Royal College of Nursing, the General Nursing Council and the Department of Health and Social Security. Thus, research in nursing could be seen to be formally accepted within the profession by identifying avenues of support for both funding and education in research methods.

From that time developments in research have been linked with developments in higher education in nursing. Since the 1970s there has been a growth in the number of academic departments of nursing in universities. Added to this more recently is the rapid expansion of nursing departments within polytechnics. Both these developments have served to promote and support research in nursing practice today, creating an increased research awareness in nursing to the extent that it is now common practice on all nurse education programmes to include research studies as part of their basic curriculum. In addition teachers are practising from a more research-aware stance and information shared with students is more likely to have a firm foundation of nursing knowledge than practices that were previously accepted without question. This latter point indicates the need for research. Nurses have recognised that poor academic preparation is no longer acceptable in the world of twentieth century health care. Practices based on ritual or tradition are acceptable only if they have a proven knowledge base to support the actions taken.

Who can do nursing research?

The answer to this question is any nurse, at any level of practice. Throughout this text, applied examples will be related to many areas of practice to illustrate the points made. No single group of nurses is confined to their area of interest. Research in nursing includes the broad areas of practice, management and education. There are jobs in nursing in which research is picked out as a key area of responsibility. Increasingly, however, a research component is being included in many nursing job descriptions. The practitioner, be she in nursing, health visiting or midwifery, is well placed to carry out clinical care research projects. The nurse manager may choose to vary the emphasis in any research into care and consider the effects of any research-based changes in managing the unit. Finally, the nurse teacher may be more interested in examining the impact of her teaching on the quality of care produced by student nurses. These examples indicate very briefly the range of subject areas that could be incorporated under the title of nursing research. Add to this the study of nursing itself, which has provided a focus for many other disciplines, such as sociology and psychology, and the area of research in nursing becomes even wider.

Summary

This chapter has briefly explored definitions of research and in so doing has stressed the importance of taking a logical planned approach to the pursuit of knowledge. In exploring the question of why we need nursing research a historical overview has been given in an attempt to illustrate why research has not always been a fundamental requisite in nursing practice. Finally, the issue of who can carry out nursing research has been briefly addressed. It has been noted that the use of research-based practices are essential for all practitioners. For those who wish to undertake studies the emphasis given to research may differ according to their role, whether it be in clinical practice, management or education.

Further reading

Abel-Smith, B. (1960) *A History of the Nursing Profession*, Heinemann, London.
Altshul, A. (1984) 'The development of research in nursing', in Cormack D.F.S. (ed.) *The Research Process in Nursing*, Blackwell Scientific, Oxford.
Davies, C. (ed.) (1980) *Rewriting Nursing History*, Croom Helm, London.
Hicks, C. (1990) *Research and Statistics: A practical introduction for nurses*, Prentice Hall, Hemel Hempstead.
Hockey, L. (1985) *Nursing Research: Mistakes and misconceptions*, Churchill Livingstone, Edinburgh.
Maggs, C. (1985) *The Origins of General Nursing*, Croom Helm, London.
Parry, N. and Parry, J. (1976) *The Rise of the Medical Profession*, Biddles Ltd, Guildford, Surrey.
Reid, N.G. and Boore, J.R.P. (1987) *Research Methods and Statistics in Health Care*, Edward Arnold, London.
Sheahan, J. (1986) 'Nursing research in Britain: The state of the art', *Nurse Education Today*, **6**, 3–10.
Smith, J. (1986) 'The end of the beginning', *Senior Nurse*, **5**(1), 14–15.

2   Research awareness

This chapter has been included to explore some of the general issues that have an impact on the ability of nurses to use research in their practice. In placing the emphasis on research awareness at this early stage in the book it is hoped that readers will realise that research-based practice is not just about doing research; it is also about being aware of the availability of research and utilising research-based knowledge in practice at every opportunity.

Research awareness

The term 'research awareness' is frequently used to denote what some may see as a special kind of skill. In fact, it is a useful term to cover all levels of interest in nursing research. Although not all nurses will be researchers all should be aware of research and have sufficient knowledge of this to utilise research in their practice.

To be aware of research implies that the practitioner has an understanding of the principles of research and has sufficient knowledge to read and critically analyse research reports. Research awareness means being prepared to question and to look for answers. It also means that the practitioner knows about the research that has been carried out in her own area of nursing and utilises that knowledge in planning or managing her practice.

In summary, research awareness means that the nurse has an insight into the research process, is questioning in her approach, is familiar with research relevant to her practice and uses that knowledge in her work.

Factors affecting research awareness

There are several reasons why research may be seen to be something separate from, rather than an integral part of, everyday nursing practice. These are explored briefly below.

Historical factors

The first reason for limited awareness of research among nurses is historical in nature. Some aspects of the historical development of nursing have been outlined in Chapter 1 and could be usefully reviewed further in relation to research awareness. One area that may be seen to have a direct bearing on the development of research awareness in nursing is linked to the close liaison of nursing to medical practice. As organised nursing developed in the UK in the nineteenth century the largely female nursing profession was in a position to observe, as medical colleagues developed their knowledge base. The development of medical knowledge was largely research-based as data was gathered in relation to a large range of treatments in both medical and surgical care. New drugs and new surgical techniques were tried and tested before any doctor could say with confidence that the prescription for care would work. In contrast, nurses were developing skill in caring based rather more on intuition and the organisation of work, in a way that has subsequently been described as a traditional approach to practice.

The end result of this is that, whereas the medical profession can trace the origins of their research back several hundred years, the evolution of nursing research in the UK has a much more recent history dating back to the 1950s and early 1960s. Nurses were not unused to research prior to that time; rather, they were accustomed to their medical colleagues undertaking research and so saw this as something separate from nursing practice. Nurses did, and still do, participate in medical research but the capacity in which this is done is more often that of a research assistant than as the initiator of research ideas. For example, nurses may distribute drugs prescribed for a medical trial or collect specimens for analysis.

It is important, however, that the liaison with medical practice is not seen as the sole reason for the failure of nurses to develop research awareness at an earlier stage in the evolution of the profession. Other factors outlined below have had an impact and will be explored in relation to this.

Nursing and intuition

It has been suggested that to be a 'good nurse' simply requires intuitive skills and a desire to help and care for others. This association can be retraced to the origins of nursing and the perceived nurturing role of the nurse. Many nurses still practice to traditional value systems in which intuition rather than sound, factual knowledge form the basis of practice. This must not be condemned outright, for there may be some areas of intuitive nursing practice that, if subject to critical scrutiny by research, would be supported as fact. However, there are perhaps other areas that would fail a 'research test'. Approaches to nursing care that are planned in a particular way for the simple reason that they have always been done that way are open to question. Many practitioners may be confident about the value of intuition in nursing, for their instinct may have guided them through many difficult situations in nursing care.

Research does not deny the individual instincts that nurses have developed in the course of their careers; rather, it seeks to identify the foundation of that intuition so that the knowledge base for practice can be clarified. It must be acknowledged that because something has always worked in a particular way before does not mean that it will always work in that way on every occasion. For example, a car driver will have had the experience of assuming that when she turns the key in the ignition the engine will start. This may be the case on most occasions but one day the expected response may not occur: the key is turned and nothing happens. If the driver has some knowledge of mechanics she may be able to work out systematically what she feels is wrong with the car and perhaps be able to fix the fault herself. If she is not able to do this she may have to call in specialist help.

To use this as an analogy it may be suggested that the nursing practitioner finds that on most occasions a given form of nursing care, based on intuition, works for her patients. However, on one occasion the expected response does not occur. If this nurse has a sound knowledge base she may review the alternatives, look for a solution to this particular problem and solve it for herself. If she does not have the appropriate knowledge then the subsequent result may be a wrong solution, which may mean that the patient does not receive the appropriate care for their problem. Unfortunately, the nurse may not be in a position to call in the rescue services, as any one of us would be if our car broke down. There may be experts at hand in the form of clinical nurse specialists who have developed a research-based approach to their work. However, the nurse who has always relied on her own intuition may treat with mistrust those nurses who have a role that is not conducive to traditional practice in nursing. Consequently, she may not be prepared to call for further advice at a time of need.

One way in which it is possible for nurses to explore the level of intuition in their own practice is to stop and ask themselves why they are carrying out care in a particular fashion. This is certainly a better way of approaching care than waiting for something to go wrong before seeking help. Also, as noted above, questioning practice serves to enhance research awareness and may facilitate the nurse in identifying a clearly defined knowledge base to her work.

Nursing and common sense

Common sense is a term that is frequently used to try to explain why we do something (or perhaps more frequently to question why someone else did not do something). There is an assumption that, in many instances, the way in which things are done reflects a common bonding of ideas and approaches to a problem, and that the subsequent method used to solve it will be common to all. We all think we know what common sense means but unfortunately, as with many other aspects of life, what we think it means and what others think it means is not always the same. In other words, common sense is not so common. Consequently, assumptions that nursing care should be based on common sense are questionable, for they can put the patient at risk.

It is appropriate to consider how nurses gain knowledge of research as a subject for, although there is a growing awareness of nursing research generally, there are still many aspects that cause concern to nurses interested in the utilisation of research findings.

Research and knowledge of research

As noted above the history of nursing research is relatively recent in the UK, covering a span of approximately 30 years. This has had an impact on the development of knowledge of research in nursing practice.

Traditional patterns of nurse education did not prepare nurses to be questioning and critical in their approach and, for many years, the role of the nurse did not come under critical scrutiny. In leading a more questioning approach to practice the efforts of the early nurse researchers were important in that nurses began to scrutinise what was happening in their profession. This in turn eventually contributed towards a redirection in nurse education, although it was to take some years before research studies were introduced into pre-registration curricula. For a long time the subject of research in nursing remained distant from its everyday practice for the majority of practitioners while research knowledge was transmitted from institutes of higher education through to post-basic courses in schools of nursing and, ultimately, to pre-registration courses. The time taken for this cascade of research knowledge to reach basic nurse education serves to explain why so many qualified practitioners remain uncertain about utilising research in their work.

Students working towards registration in schools of nursing represent the majority of nurses in this country. They are now commonly introduced to research methods in their basic courses, but it must be stressed this is only a recent innovation. The introduction of a research-orientated approach in nurse education has been a slow process.

The key people involved in teaching research are, of course, the nurse teachers. There are many teachers of nursing who themselves had to learn about research before they could confidently teach the subject to students. Many of these teachers were themselves educated in the traditional mode in which research as a subject was not part of the syllabus.

Two further issues can be seen as directly linked with education. These are the ability of nurses to understand the research information presented to them and the wider issue of its availability.

Understanding research

The ability of nurses to understand research links directly with education, for if this is inadequate then they will continue to have difficulty in understanding its purpose and value. It must be acknowledged that, although there are increasing numbers of nurses studying research, either through formal courses or self-directed study, there is still a need to consider ways in which their individual understanding can be enhanced.

One area that is frequently cited as causing a difficulty to nurses is the style of presentation of research reports. Frequently, the presentation of information does not meet the needs of those people for whom it is intended – that is, the rank and file of practising nurses. Several reasons are seen as contributing to this.

The use of 'jargon' is commonly noted as a factor that makes it difficult to understand research reports. This is not an intentional ploy on the part of the researchers, rather it indicates that very often published research has been undertaken as part of an academic study. The language used commonly reflects the requirement at that level but, while easily understood by those initiated into the rigours of academic life, it is not so comprehensible to those who have not had similar experience. Researchers themselves are well aware of this problem and some attempt to overcome it by writing their reports in two formats: the first for academic presentation, the second a summarised version for a more general readership. Some people may disagree with researchers taking a dual approach when presenting their research findings and argue that if the standard of research is to be maintained, then the type of presentation should be consistent. However, if more nurses are to become aware of research it is crucial that every opportunity is used to share knowledge in a way that the majority of practitioners can understand.

Another aspect that frequently acts as a deterrent to nurses reading research reports is the use of statistical tables. As will be seen in Chapter 8, the use of statistical data in research reports is to support and explain the information given by the researcher in the text. Nurses need have only an elementary knowledge of statistics to find the inclusion of this data beneficial when reading research reports.

Availability of research

The discussion above appears to presume the availability of research. Before examining this aspect it will be useful to review issues related to library services that may impinge on its availability to nurses.

Access to a good library is crucial if research awareness in nurses is to be developed. In some schools of nursing in the past the library resources available were extremely limited and did not carry the necessary texts to enhance the understanding of research. This factor has been recognised and many centres are now developing excellent library resources for nurses. Issues that librarians have had to consider include not only the resources available but also how to offer a flexible service to meet the needs of nurses in their area. This is important, for nurses, as a group, are disparate in both their knowledge base and their ability to match their working hours to the opening hours of the library. Many initiatives are taking place at a local level in an attempt to meet these needs. Flexible opening hours is one example that can be used to illustrate this point. All newcomers to nursing research would be well advised to familiarise themselves with their local library and to use the skills offered by the librarian when developing their knowledge base. In addition to the local library there are other library resources available; these are discussed in more detail in Chapter 6.

It is quite feasible that the nurse may seek out the literature relating to research in a given subject area only to find that its availability is rather limited. Although there is a growing amount of nursing research available the volume does not necessarily meet the needs of all nurses. The research may be plentiful in total but, when focusing onto a specific subject area, there may in fact be a dearth of information. For example, in picking up a nursing index to identify any relevant research studies the newcomer may be impressed by the volume of work undertaken and feel initially optimistic about finding work done in relation to her own speciality. However, if she works in a specialist field she may find it difficult to identify work specifically related to the subject. A good illustration of this would be to consider the rise in 'new' specialities in nursing over recent years. It may be a few years before the nurse working in a transplant unit is able to identify a good volume of nursing research that is specific to her area of practice. Although there may be relevant studies undertaken into more general aspects of nursing care, in the early days of new treatments it is the pioneers of the speciality who have the responsibility of establishing the knowledge base. The situation is further complicated by the fact that, because of the stage of development of nursing research, many reported studies are only small-scale and cannot be said to generalise to all situations. There is an undoubted need to replicate studies in a variety of settings to test the adequacy of the findings in a broader setting, but this aspect is only developing in line with the pace of development of nursing research in general. This may cause frustration for the nurse trying to find research into her area of interest. To attempt to change practice on the basis of findings from an inadequate research study could result in unsafe practices in care.

Applying research

Research, quite commonly, generates more questions than answers. Thus, the nurse seeking information to help in her work may still find herself faced with a number of questions rather than a clearly defined action plan for applying research.

A criticism that could be directed at experimental research, for example, may be that the studies themselves are carried out in such a manner that they do not reflect the day-to-day practice of nursing. Researchers are able to manipulate the variables in a way that may be beyond the control of practising nurses. For example, much research work is undertaken into communication in patient care in hospital. Depending upon the research design the researcher may have been able to control the time spent in communicating with the patients. Consequently, although the result of such a study may demonstrate the importance of spending time communicating with patients, the nurse working in a busy ward may not be able to utilise the research for the simple reason that her unit is short of staff. The nurse in the ward or unit may have less time available to her than that allocated to nurse–patient communication by the researcher.

However, the nurse can still use the research in a constructive way. She may be able to use the findings to make a case for more staff in her unit and therefore work towards creating the right environment in which these findings can be utilised. Consequently, although at the outset some research may be seen to reflect an ideal environment, it can still have utility value in practice. Some issues related to use of research in practice are discussed in Chapter 10.

Cost of research

The subject of funding research studies will be discussed further in Chapter 4, but it has been included here to indicate that there are cost implications in preparing nurses to be aware of research. If we are to provide opportunity for nurses to study research we should consider the costs involved. Not only would teaching time need to be considered but also the costs of releasing nurses from their area of practice in order to undertake their studies. Costs will vary depending on the time spent in study, which can range in time from short study sessions over a few hours to weeks or months on a more in-depth course.

Disseminating research findings

Unless the results of research are shared it is unlikely that research-based nursing practice will advance much further. The first issue that will be addressed in relation to this is who is responsible for disseminating research findings. Secondly, ways of doing this will be discussed.

Who is responsible for disseminating research?

All nurses hold responsibility for ensuring that their practice is based on sound knowledge. Consequently, all practitioners should be involved in the dissemination of research findings. It will be useful to consider this further in relation to the specific roles of the researcher, the manager and the teacher in nursing.

The researcher

Planning for research should include consideration of how findings from the completed study should be disseminated to the profession. This is important not only from the point of view of sharing the findings from a specific project, but also as a means of stimulating and maintaining the interest of nurses who have not had the opportunity of studying research.

The nurse researcher is obviously the key person in terms of ensuring that any research findings are disseminated to the profession. However, not all researchers in nursing are employed purely as research workers and this has implications for the dissemination of findings. A nurse may, for example, undertake a research project as part of an advanced course of study. If she is employed full time in a clinical post she may not be in a position to go out and meet other nurses to share her research findings with them. However willing she is to do this her employers may not be able to release her for the time required to do this effectively. Despite this, the nurse who has a locally based research post may find it easier to share information with colleagues than one who is undertaking research at a national level as part of an advanced course of study.

The research method adopted may play a part in facilitating feedback to the profession. Methods which involve research nurses working alongside their colleagues can be a useful means of disseminating research findings. For example, participant observation techniques are one means by which researchers and practitioners can work alongside each other, perhaps developing a rapport which facilitates dissemination of findings once the study is complete. Action research is another method in which the researcher may work closely with staff involved with the study (see Chapter 7).

Although in an ideal world it should be the researcher who takes the initiative in disseminating research knowledge, this may not always be feasible and other means of filtering information through to practising nurses must be considered.

The nurse manager

In a world in which managerial accountability is emphasised the importance of research to nurse managers cannot be underestimated. The manager is ideally placed to be the link between the researcher and the practitioner. If the researcher shares her findings with a ward sister then that sister may effect a change in practice as appropriate within her unit. If the researcher shares her findings with a manager then the cascade effect of sharing information may result in dissemination of findings to several units that are the responsibility of the manager.

The teacher

The teacher in nursing is commonly seen as a resource for knowledge and this is as true in the area of research as in other aspects of nursing practice. Teachers have responsibility for sharing research knowledge with two groups: student nurses, at pre- and post-registration level, and practitioners working in clinical areas. Consequently, the teacher role is crucial when considering the dissemination of research findings. The impact of a lively, well-prepared lecture or discussion on the subject of research has the potential of effecting a critical review of practice in many areas.

Quite commonly, the teacher carries much responsibility for sustaining an interest in research once it has been generated. Once a research-based approach to education has been adopted it is important to maintain the initiative and not revert to traditional patterns of education.

How can research findings be disseminated?

There are several ways in which research findings can be disseminated and for the purpose of clarity they will be discussed under separate headings.

Returning information to the research site

When researchers seek permission to undertake research they commonly make a promise to let those people who have participated in the study know of the results as soon as they are made available. This can be a very useful way of sharing research findings; the interest of participants is likely to be high because of personal involvement in the research. An additional benefit is that insight gained from participants after the event might be useful to the researcher in planning future studies. For example, the sample group may wish to make observations about their perception of research methods used in the study. It is important that researchers recognise these factors and ensure that they share their findings through these channels. Another reason that this is important is in considering the interests of future studies being undertaken within that environment. If staff receive promises of feedback from researchers and these promises are not met they are less likely to co-operate with future researchers looking for permission to undertake studies in that area.

Publishing research findings

One of the most obvious ways to share research findings is to ensure that the results are published and shared with as many people as possible. This may seem obvious, but it does cause difficulty in practice. The first point is that the ability to write well is not a skill possessed by every nurse. Consequently, as noted in Chapter 9, although a nurse may have undertaken a good piece of research, if she does not find writing easy the project may never be completed for want of a written report.

Even if the nurse researcher has the necessary writing skills, there still remains the problem of disseminating the work through the written media. First, writing often takes a long time and newcomers to research often under-estimate the time that it will take to prepare their work for publication. A useful guide for researchers to work to is that the time allowed for writing a report should represent about a third of the total time allowed for the whole research project. If the time taken for material to be published is added to this it can be seen that there is a long time span between beginning a research project and publication.

The second problem is that there are only a limited number of national and international journals that publish nursing research. As a result of this the time taken for publication can be variable, extending in some instances to a couple of years. The immediate relevance of a research project may be lost in a time lapse such as this, so the nurse researcher needs to consider other ways of disseminating her findings. In considering quicker ways in which to communicate their findings than the national publication process researchers might be able to identify whether there are any local journals that could be used to disseminate information to nurses who might have particular interest in the study. Many health districts now have small journals for local news and comments and the editors are often looking for material to publish in these.

Study days and conferences

Study days and nursing conferences provide a useful medium for sharing experiences and consequently offer one of the most common routes for dis-seminating research findings. These forums are not confined to a select group of nurse researchers. One of the positive developments of post-basic courses in nurse education today is that students who have undertaken research studies will frequently report their findings on a locally arranged study day. Such an approach has the benefit of identifying issues specifically related to the loc-ality and can therefore be a useful means of increasing research awareness.

Research interest groups

There are a number of research interest groups in this country; they provide a means by which those people interested in research can share experiences. While providing a forum for the dissemination of findings from research studies, these groups also offer a resource for those people undertaking research. Local research interest groups may be identified within the hospital, the district or at regional level. In addition there are national research interest groups, associated with professional organisations such as the Royal College of Nursing.

Research appreciation courses

Research courses are another common way in which information can be disseminated. The nurse undertaking the course will become increasingly aware of research as the programme develops. In addition to this her colleagues may express an interest and make enquiries about the content of the course. This may ultimately motivate others to undertake research studies themselves.

Approaches to nurse education

Finally, it is worth considering briefly the part played by education in general in disseminating research findings. If the style of nurse education encourages questioning and demands that the knowledge base of practice is research-based then it is highly likely that this approach will stay with the student nurse throughout her career.

Distance learning, an important educational development, is a useful means of facilitating educational opportunity for nurses. This approach can be utilised regardless of irregular working hours and other difficulties that sometimes hinder nurses wishing to undertake advanced study and has been adopted by some centres as a means of sharing research knowledge. Further details relating to distance-learning packages for nursing research can be obtained from the Distance Learning Centre at the South Bank Polytechnic, London.

Summary

The focus of this chapter has been the subject of research awareness and an attempt has been made to provide a definition for this term. Factors that may affect the level of research awareness have been discussed. Finally, the issue of disseminating research findings has been addressed, the responsibilities held by nurses at different levels has been outlined and the various means by which experiences can be shared have been discussed.

Further reading

Flitton, D. (1984) *Nurse Researchers in the UK in 1980: Research activity in relation to area of employment*, Edinburgh University Monographs, Edinburgh.

Hunt, J. (1981) 'Indicators for practice: The use of research findings', *Journal of Advanced Nursing*, **6**, 189–94.

Lelean, S.R. (1982) 'The implementation of research findings in practice', *International Journal of Nursing Studies*, **19**(4), 223–30.

Myco, F. (1980) 'Nursing Research information. Are Nurse Educators and Practitioners seeking it out?' *Journal of Advanced Nursing*, **5**, 637–46.

3   Ideas for research

The main purpose of this chapter is to indicate how ideas for a research study may be derived. This has been included as nurses approaching research studies for the first time often have difficulty in determining how to focus their work. They might ask why things happen but, in following this query through, become diverted to other interesting areas of study. Alternatively, they may have an interest in an area of practice but are uncertain as to where to begin planning a research study. In cases such as these nurses may become diverted from an original line of enquiry and attempt to explore too many issues.

Thinking about research

The newcomer to nursing research may be faced with a barrage of questions when thinking about research. These include issues such as where researchers get their ideas, how they decide which specific aspects to research and who gives support to the newcomer to research? Other issues may include questions as to what part employers play in determining what should be researched. These aspects will be explored in more detail in the next chapter, which focuses on planning research.

Although fairly simple at first glance, it is these issues that cause anxiety to the newcomer to research. It is not uncommon for the nurse approaching research studies for the first time to feel hesitant as to which direction to take when thinking about research ideas. She may have the ideas, but be uncertain as to how to utilise them in a study of her own area of practice.

The amount of research information available is vast and unless an organised approach is taken it is too easy to become caught up in literature in such a way that the main focus of the proposed study becomes diluted. In this situation the nurse wanting to undertake research may become disheartened, for the implications of an initial study idea may become so vast as to make any proposed project seem an impossibility. The result in this situation may be an overloading of the senses to the extent that reading stops and any further interest or development of research ideas becomes stifled.

Equally, the nurse who wants to initiate research-based practice may become so immersed in a very large area of interest that she is unable to instigate any changes simply because there are too many to choose from. Consequently, she may find it difficult to be specific about which path to follow. Streamlining of ideas should help ensure a more positive outcome in both these situations.

Generating research ideas

Consideration of how research ideas can be generated will help the nurse to identify with the processes that researchers go through when undertaking projects.

Research projects can be generated from two sources. The first is from individual researchers themselves, who may have a specific area of interest which motivates them to develop their knowledge by undertaking research into the subject. The second source is that in which an organisation or employer identifies an area of need for further study and consequently may employ a researcher to undertake the necessary work. These two sources of research ideas may be closely related. For example, a nurse working in any clinical environment may feel that some aspect of care should be closely scrutinised. She may then approach her employers for permission and time to undertake a research project into this area and subsequently may be given support to do this. Alternatively, the employer may recognise a need for a particular study to be done and approach a nurse who is known to have a special interest in the topic with a request to her to undertake the work.

There are occasions when nurses undertaking courses of study in which a research project is part of the course requirement may approach their employers for guidance on which subject areas it would be useful to research. Occasionally, there are situations when employers maintain the right to choose topics for research if they are funding a member of staff through an academic course that involves a research study. It should, perhaps, also be noted that in addition to the two sources of research noted above there will be occasions when another person has the original 'idea', which is then followed up by someone else with a research interest. There are undoubtedly many 'ideas people' in our society who can inspire others to work towards achieving a goal and the value of such people is not underestimated by researchers.

For the new nurse researcher a good starting point for any research is to begin by looking at practice in the area in which she works. This has the advantage of making the research more meaningful and therefore, perhaps, helps her to maintain interest as the study becomes complex and time-consuming. The major disadvantage of this approach is that in looking at practice the nurse is faced with so many choices that it is difficult to determine exactly which aspect should be studied first.

A useful tip at this stage is to identify a 'mentor' who will help to clarify ideas. This person could save a lot of anxiety by helping to clarify ideas at an early stage in the study of research. Those people who commonly fall into the category of mentors for nurses undertaking research are those who are seen to have some knowledge of the subject, such as known research nurses, teachers or colleagues who have undertaken a research study. If the newcomer to research has difficulty in clarifying research ideas she will need to consider how to overcome this problem and one way of doing this is to use the frameworks offered in the many nursing models available to practitioners today.

Using a nursing model to generate research ideas

Sometimes an interest in research is generated when new ideas or theory relating to care are introduced. A recent development that could fall into this category is that of nursing models. In putting forward their views of nursing, theorists frequently make a plea to the profession to test their ideas in practice. Obviously, the more nurses who can do this the more the knowledge base of nursing will become established. However, there are other ways in which nursing models can be utilised by researchers.

When trying to clarify ideas it is useful to begin with a clearly defined framework that will help to structure thought processes. If this principle is applied to nursing research it is advisable to consider which frameworks are available to guide nursing practice. Following this line of thought, one 'framework' available to nurses today is the many nursing models that have been presented by nurse theorists as a means of identifying the knowledge base of nursing practice. The need for research into the use of their proposed model of nursing is frequently identified by nurse theorists. Although it is acknowledged that such research is badly needed the use of a model to help structure ideas, as described in this chapter, is at a different level in suggesting that nurses use these frameworks to help to clarify research ideas. The use of nursing models in helping to structure approaches to research would seem to be a logical development of using these frameworks to guide practice.

The model that will be used as an example in this text is the Roper *et al.* (1985) model of nursing. This has been chosen because it has been widely adopted by nurses in the British health care system and consequently is familiar to many practising nurses. In focusing on the Activities of Living (ALs) this framework provides a useful means of illustrating one way in which a nursing model can be used to help to clarify research ideas.

Table 3.1   Activities of Living (Roper *et al.*, 1985)

Maintaining a safe environment
Communicating
Breathing
Eating and drinking
Eliminating
Personal cleansing and dressing
Controlled body temperature
Mobilising
Working and playing
Expressing sexuality
Sleeping
Dying

Roper *et al.* list 12 aspects of the Activities of Living model that should be considered by nurses when assessing, planning, implementing and evaluating nursing care (Table 3.1). If this model was used to provide a framework to generate research ideas the nurse could, for example, create a grid which would help to identify aspects of care that could be a subject either for research or for creating a logical approach research-based focus for nursing practice.

The use of a grid has been developed in Table 3.2. Each activity of living is identified and alongside this is a subject area that could be developed into a research idea. Some of these areas can be seen to be physiological in nature, while others have a more psychological or sociological orientation. This is an important point to note, for it reinforces the wide-ranging areas open to those wishing to undertake research in nursing. The use of this grid is also helpful in that it demonstrates how a subject area can be reduced to component parts. A nurse may start with an interest in research in which she states that her study will be into the area of communication in nursing. One glance at the grid shows that, even with just a preliminary outline, this subject is too vast to explore as a whole. The nurse must be much more specific in her stated aim. The art of being specific and concise in stating the aims of a research study is one that develops with experience in research. Generally, it may be noted that the more precise a researcher is in defining the boundaries of a study the more likely she is to produce a valuable piece of work successfully. The newcomer to research can often flounder in her study, for lack of precision can result in lack of direction or, more commonly, may mean that the topic is too big to study properly. This issue is discussed further in subsequent chapters.

The list in Table 3.2 is by no means conclusive and, if drawn up by another writer, could show quite a different pattern. However, Table 3.2 indicates a number of areas that could be explored from such differing perspectives as management, education or clinical practice. The emphasis given

Table 3.2 Framework for research ideas

Activities of Living (Roper et al., 1985)	Areas for research
Maintaining a safe environment	Accidents – hospital/home Falls in the elderly Equipment safety
Communicating	Nurse/patient Nurse/nurse Patient/client anxiety Patient understanding
Breathing	Anxiety Smoking habits – patients – nurses Equipment and aids
Eating and drinking	Quality of diet Monitoring intake Accuracy of recordings Analysis of statements e.g., 'encourage fluids'
Elimination	Incontinence – causes – effects – aids Toilet facilities Catheter care
Personal cleansing and dressing	Ability to care Care meeting needs Clothing available Hygiene standards and risks
Controlling body temperature	Methods of recording Accuracy of recording Necessity of recordings
Mobilising	Assessing ability Aids required Evaluating aids used
Working and playing	Home care facilities Cultural needs Employment and health
Expressing sexuality	Meeting individual needs Attitudes to patients Body image
Sleeping	Sleeping patterns – in hospital – on night duty Physiology of sleep
Dying	Care in hospital Care in the community Communication issues Support for relatives

to any subsequent study would vary according to the specific interests of the researcher.

To illustrate the points made above it might be useful to review some examples. If we begin with an example with a clinical orientation it can be seen that alongside the AL 'Controlling Body Temperature' the research idea noted is that of recording a patient's temperature. This is a common activity for nurses working in a variety of settings and is an important aspect of monitoring physiological activity of the body. A clinical nurse may be interested in identifying whether any research has been done into the accuracy of recording temperatures in clinical areas. She may choose to compare the accuracy of mercurial thermometers with electrical thermometers with a view to changing the approach in that clinical area. The nurse manager may develop the idea rather differently and choose to investigate the cost implications of nurses routinely taking temperature recordings. Although not labelled as acutely ill, patients may be subject to the 'routine' of temperature-taking simply because it is part of normal ward activity and therefore incorporated into all planned care. This may not cause the individual any stress, but the nurse manager is more concerned in this study with the effective use of nursing time. If temperature recording is not required it could be seen as a waste of nursing time, an important consideration in times of economic stringency.

The nurse teacher might approach this topic from yet another angle. From an educational perspective she might have an interest in the subject of the theory–practice gap, an expression used to illustrate what may be perceived as a discrepancy between what nursing students are taught in schools of nursing and what is practised in clinical areas. To ensure that there is continuity between theory and practice it is not only important that correct, research-based techniques are taught to students but that these skills are practised correctly in clinical areas. Consequently, the nurse teacher may choose to study how the skills required to take temperatures are utilised in the ward areas.

An example with a *psychological orientation* in the research areas listed in Table 3.2 can be found alongside the AL 'Communicating'. It is worth noting that much nursing research has been done in the area of communication and this work provides relevant reading for all nurses. Awareness of research work that has been done may help to increase utilisation of these studies in practice. The nurse in the surgical ward might have a specific interest in preparing people psychologically for the surgical procedures that they are about to face. The nurse manager of a unit might be more interested in exploring communication between ward nurses and relatives of patients who are in hospital. This interest might, for example, have been generated as a result of a series of complaints from a patient's relatives. The nurse teacher might be interested in communication from the point of view of preparing student nurses to communicate effectively with those people for whom they are caring.

Research with a *sociological orientation* can be identified under the AL 'Working and Playing'. For example, the facilities available in the community for people who have suffered a cerebro-vascular accident will be of interest to nurses in hospital and the community. The district nurse might be looking at this topic from the perspective of a direct care-giver. The nurse manager might be considering how best to facilitate the care given by ensuring provision of appropriate resources. The nurse teacher would be interested from the point of view of ensuring that students are able to work with community staff in an environment in which good quality care is facilitated by the provision of appropriate support to learner nurses.

It is worth restating that the research areas noted in Table 3.2 are simply prompts towards developing research ideas. The general subject areas noted could provide the focus for developing ideas for a more in-depth study.

Summary

In summary, this chapter has outlined some areas from which research ideas could be generated. Without a clearly defined framework much time and energy can be wasted in trying to clarify research ideas. Consequently, it has been recommended that potential nurse researchers use the nursing models available to provide a structure by which research ideas can be categorised and refined into clear statements of intent. To illustrate this point the Roper *et al.* (1980) model based on the Activities of Living has been used in this chapter. This approach is just one idea as to how to generate research ideas and identify clearly defined areas for study.

Further reading

Aggleton, P. and Chalmers, H. (1986) *Nursing Models and The Nursing Process,* Macmillan Education, London.
Darling, V.H. and Rogers, J. (1986) *Research for Practising Nurses,* Macmillan Education, London.
George, J.B. (ed.) (1985) *Nursing Theories: The base for professional practice,* Prentice Hall, Hemel Hempstead.
Redfern, S. (1984) 'Asking the research question', in Cormack, D.F.S. *The Research Process in Nursing,* Blackwell Scientific, Oxford.
Roper, W., Logan, N. and Tierney, A. (1985) *The Elements of Nursing,* Churchill Livingstone, Edinburgh.

4   Planning a research project

This chapter outlines some of the practical issues that should be considered when planning a research project. Research projects of any sort make heavy demands on the researcher; also, the nature of research often means that risks must be taken and there may be times when plans do not develop as desired. All recruits to nursing research should be aware of these factors so that they use time and energy well throughout the study and recognise that there will be times of despondency, as well as times of satisfaction when all appears to be going to plan.

Planning for research

The importance of planning cannot be underestimated in any research project. Careful planning at all stages will not only help towards achieving a better quality research study but, more importantly from the researcher's point of view, it will save much time and effort as the study progresses. When decorating a room colour schemes are planned and the surfaces carefully prepared for a new coat of paint. The benefits of this are obvious to any experienced decorator. The results of careful planning and preparation are that in anticipating what needs to be done in the early stages delays are avoided, all the necessary equipment is at hand and the quality of the end result reflects the planning and preparation.

So it is with the nurse researcher. Careful consideration of all the issues involved and a plan that is well structured and logical in relation to all aspects of the research process can help to avoid problems as the study is developed and enhance the quality of the completed work.

Factors to consider when planning research

The first, and seemingly obvious, factor that the nurse researcher must consider is *what* it is that she wishes to research.

Defining the problem area may seem to be a very simple step to take but, as noted in Chapter 3, deciding what to research is often the most difficult aspect of planning research. For example, a nurse may have a project in mind relating to stress and cancer. In planning this she may feel that such a topic is suitable for research and, perhaps, be considering how to identify the type of stressors in life that may contribute towards the development of cancer. However, this nurse needs to ask herself more questions, the first of which is whether the *subject is researchable*. The original idea noted above of studying types of stress that may contribute towards cancer development is potentially a good one but the implications of undertaking such a study are enormous. This can usefully be explored further in relation to the points noted below which are considered to be important factors when planning to undertake research in nursing.

Outlining the problem area

At the outset all the concepts used within research studies should be spelt out and all boundaries clearly defined. When clarifying the area of research the questions that should be asked in relation to the example given above include defining concepts such as 'stress', and clarifying exactly what this means in the context of the research. If the nurse is going to look at this in terms of all the stress that occurs in life she will have to make a very long list to give a fully comprehensive picture of what is meant by this term.

Coupled with this is the need to set the boundaries of the research by stating which type of 'cancer' is going to provide the focus of the study. If she plans to study the subject of stress and its effects on all types of cancer the boundaries of this project are enormous and perhaps unrealistic for a single researcher. Consequently, defining a realistic problem area is a crucial step when planning a research study. This subject will be considered further in the next chapter.

Time available

Nurses who undertake research for the first time often do not appreciate how time-consuming it is to carry out a well-planned research project. As a result they can become very frustrated with the work while it is in progress simply because of pressures on time. Consequently, the nurse researcher needs to consider how much *time* is available to her to undertake her project. Obviously, if she was about to embark on a full-time research project covering a time span of several years then the boundaries of her study will be far greater than that of a nurse planning a three-month project while allocated to a surgical unit.

While the nurse embarking on a full-time study may be able to develop her original ideas to explore any possible links between stress in life and the development of cancer, the nurse in the second category noted above will have to determine a research question that can be studied effectively in the limited time available. As a result the focus of the study may change to reflect this. For example, instead of looking at stress and the link with cancer from a cause and effect point of view, she may change the emphasis in her research problem to review the type of stress that a diagnosis of cancer would cause in an individual. It is not uncommon for researchers to modify their initial ideas in this way to come up with a research study that is feasible in the time available.

Research experience

The *experience* of the nurse researcher is another factor that will have an effect when planning research. Newcomers to research may be advised to start with a simple project first. Many experienced researchers can identify the difficulties they encountered in undertaking their first research studies and will note the value of learning the pitfalls of research before getting involved in a major project. The research process is not learned from reading textbooks; it is best learned by doing. In 'doing' research a great deal of insight can be gained that cannot be gathered from a book, however widely read the individual. In doing a small-scale study researchers may not be able to generalise the findings to a variety of settings but this does not mean that the work will have no value. Many small-scale research projects have had considerable practical use at a local level. Moreover, if a number of small-scale studies are replicated and the same results identified, ultimately it may be possible to generalise findings based on cumulative evidence.

Financial implications

The financial implications of research should always be considered at an early stage of planning for research. At a very basic level researchers need to consider that time costs money so, even if a nurse is undertaking a small research project in her own unit, there is an initial cost implication based on the time allocated for undertaking the research. This point is not made to discourage research being undertaken during working hours but rather to emphasise that no research project is free of financial consideration. Nurse researchers involved in large-scale projects are well aware of the cost of time, for they may have to make a case for research assistants to help in undertaking the work involved in a research study. In doing this they need to calculate salary costs for the assistant, and perhaps associated secretarial support that may be required throughout a study.

It is also important to consider the cost in relation to the time spent by respondents when participating in the study. Admittedly, this may be a hidden cost, but researchers need to be aware of this when planning research projects for it may affect the willingness of people to participate in the study. For example, if a number of nurses in a clinical unit were asked to participate in an interview lasting one hour the time involved could be extensive.

Those aspects of research that may involve direct financial outlay include preparation of materials required for data collection, for example, the typing costs if a questionnaire is to be used. As noted in Chapter 7, the presentation of questionnaires may effect the response rate so this is an important point to consider; every effort should be made to produce a well-designed questionnaire. The cost of copying questionnaires for circulation is also important, as is the cost of postage if that is the chosen method of circulation. Finally, the costs involved in the typing and presentation of research reports is another most important consideration as this can be extremely expensive, particularly for large-scale projects. Other miscellaneous costs that may need to be considered include travelling expenses and any other equipment necessary to the study. The researcher undertaking a qualitative study may, for example, require a tape recorder with which to record interviews with the population being studied.

Funding research

Although quite a lot of small-scale research in nursing is carried out without application for funds some source of funding may be necessary to undertake more complex studies. The amount of financial support sought through funding agencies can vary from small sums that will help to offset the costs of producing a research tool to full funding which includes paying salaries for the researchers and their assistants, in addition to all other anticipated expenditure.

The sources of funding for research are varied and can range from the employer to national bodies in both a professional and voluntary capacity. The demand for funds for research may exceed the resources available; therefore, the researcher may need to spend a certain amount of time and energy in the search for funding. Nursing libraries commonly stock directories of charitable organisations that may be approached with applications for research funds. Further advice on this can be sought from senior nurses in the district, professional bodies within the health service and those professional organisations to which nurses belong.

Supervisor/mentor support

Experienced researchers will know of the value of having a research super-visor to advise and guide their progress through more complex studies. A supervisor will offer support and advice to a researcher undertaking a project and, more importantly, they may help to save time by helping to avoid any of those errors that frustrate researchers in moments of crisis throughout any research project. As noted in Chapter 3, it is advisable to identify a mentor from the outset when clarifying areas for research, as advice at this point can help to avoid frustration in the early stages of a study.

Nurses undertaking research as part of an academic course of study will usually have a supervisor identified as they begin their work. However, nurses working in clinical areas wishing to undertake research may have to look around to identify a suitable person for this role. This may be a colleague who has had some experience of doing research themselves or a more senior member of staff who feels able to guide and give support and advice when required. If there is no one in the immediate work environment to give support of this nature then a review of personnel working in the district might identify people who can act in a supervisory capacity. For example, there may be someone in the school of nursing who has a research interest. Alternatively, the district may have a research nurse employed to review differing aspects of nursing care.

In addition, there may be an active nursing research interest group avail-able locally. Members of such groups are generally supportive towards each other when developing research projects and so may be helpful in identifying resources.

Nursing management and research

At this point it is worth considering briefly the role of nursing management in monitoring research activities in nursing. It is essential that a clearly defined policy is available, giving guidelines about the procedures involved in under-taking research within each district. Nurse managers are responsible for pre-paring such policies and making them available to nursing staff.

The formality involved in seeking permission for research may vary. It may be sufficient for the manager to state that it is acceptable for the study to proceed as long as those people directly involved are approached and permis-sion for participation obtained directly from them. For example, a nurse may wish to study methods of work in her own unit as part of her own learning of the research process. The permission of the ward or unit manager may be all that is required to do this. If the nurse manager feels that the implications of such a study extend beyond that ward or unit they may advise the potential researcher to seek permission to undertake their research through more formal channels. It is important to stress that there are many local variations in this, so any nurse intending to carry out research should clarify the local procedures for seeking permission before proceeding. From an ethical, and purely courteous, perspective no nurse should undertake a research project without discussing it first with the nursing managers concerned.

There will be occasions when the nurse does not wish to liaise directly with the immediate manager in the unit to be studied for fear of introducing bias into the study. For example, if the nurse researcher wished to monitor ways in which work was organised in a unit it is possible that the approach to work might change as a result of her observations if staff knew they were being monitored. (The reasons for this are discussed more fully in Chapter 7.) Consequently, each case has to be considered in detail and the level at which permission for the research is sought from nursing management should match the requirements for the study.

Another aspect related to nursing management is that of gaining the co-operation of all those other people who may be directly or indirectly involved with the research. Many projects have succeeded only because co-operation was willingly given; the acknowledgements printed in most research papers serve to reinforce this point. Co-operation from all participants is like a tonic to the researcher; lack of support at times of need can result in despondency and frustration.

When reading research projects it can be seen that it is standard practice for researchers to make note of how permission to undertake the project was obtained.

Ethical issues

One of the major difficulties facing researchers is in determining when it is acceptable to continue with the study in hand and when it should be discontinued because the work transcends the boundaries of what may be considered acceptable from an ethical point of view. A research supervisor should be in a position to give an objective view on this aspect of any proposed study. Indeed, the value of having a good supervisor is that they would not allow a nurse to proceed with any study likely to have major ethical implications or cause undue suffering to anyone participating in the research.

As knowledge of nursing research increases nurses are becoming more skilled at determining which areas of study may engender ethical dilemmas. It may be useful to explore the example used earlier to illustrate the complexity of making decisions about proceeding with research projects. A nurse on a surgical unit may wish to study the stress that a diagnosis of cancer may bring to her patients. Given that they may have only just been told of the diagnosis the patient is bound to be very distressed. To ask this person to participate in a research study at this time may create additional suffering. To add to the distress of the individual would be in direct conflict with the purpose of research which, in the pursuit of knowledge, is aiming to alleviate suffering wherever possible. Consequently, the format of the proposed study should be critically and sensitively planned to ensure that no additional suffering occurs.

The way in which it is proposed that the study is carried out is relevant to these ethical dilemmas. For example, distress may occur if an approach is adopted in which the researcher, with a clipboard in hand, asks the patient direct questions from a structured questionnaire about the 'stress' they are experiencing. The nature of the subject under review lends itself to a more subtle approach in determining the patient's reactions to the condition. Informal interviews are an alternative that may be utilised, for conversational techniques may be less stressful than the rigid format of a structured interview.

The timing of the study is another consideration. Although the researcher may want to identify the initial reaction of the patient it may be better to undertake such work at a later date. This means that the information is gathered after the event and is based on recall rather than the 'here and now'. This technique of gathering data retrospectively is commonly used in research.

Although the approaches outlined above reflect differences in research methodology, what is at issue here is not the research method but the effect that different approaches to research may have on the individual being studied. It is essential that the researcher considers all these factors from an ethical point of view when planning research projects.

Ethical Committees

It is recognised that there are occasions when researchers, in their pursuit of knowledge, may face ethical dilemmas when determining the boundaries of their study. To ensure that the interests and safety of the public are maintained it is important that an external agency monitors the work of researchers. Ethical Committees are a well-established means of doing this in all health districts. The purpose of these committees is to ensure that any research undertaken, involving members of the general public in particular, is not of itself likely to cause any degree of distress or harm to those individuals participating in the study. In the past these committees, based at district and regional level, have dealt primarily with applications for medical research but now, as the level of research knowledge increases, the number of applications for nursing research taken to these committees is increasing. It should be noted that some health districts have specific approval mechanisms for nursing research that is undertaken on a small scale. This is usually co-ordinated through the nursing management structure. If these groups feel that it is pertinent to do so they will advise the nurse to take her research proposals to the district ethical committees. Because of local variations it is essential that the nurse clarifies the approvals system within her own health district before embarking on any data collection as part of her research.

Data Protection Act

There is one more aspect that should be noted following discussion on ethical issues in research. This is related to the right of individuals to privacy in terms of information that is made publicly available to them. The Data Protection Act is designed to protect those individual rights. It has important implications for researchers both from the point of view of collecting information and in writing information in research reports. The details of the Act are complex and beyond the scope of this book. A series of booklets produced by the Data Protection Registrar have been written to inform individuals of their rights under this Act. The eight guidelines produced in the series are listed in the further reading section at the end of the chapter.

Research proposal

An important aspect of preparing for research is for the researcher to write out a clearly defined plan of action, known as a research proposal. This offers the benefit of giving the researcher a structure or framework to work to when going through the research process. In addition, if the researcher is seeking permission from an Ethical Committee to undertake a project and is searching for funds to finance the study a research proposal is required. This is important for the committees concerned to be able to make an objective judgement as to the value, or otherwise, of the proposed study. There is further information about writing research proposals in Chapter 9.

Summary

In summary, this chapter has explored some of the factors that must be considered by nurses planning to undertake research projects. Specific areas addressed include defining the problem area, managing time, financial and ethical issues. Consideration of these wide-ranging issues should help to avoid complications as the research study develops.

Further reading

Cormack, D.F.S. (1984) *The Research Process in Nursing*, Blackwell Scientific, Oxford.

Data Protection Registrar (March 1987, Revised)
  Guideline 1: Introduction to the Act
  Guideline 2: The Definitions
  Guideline 3: The Register and Registration
  Guideline 4: The Data Protection Principles
  Guideline 5: Individual Rights
  Guideline 6: The Exemptions
  Guideline 7: Enforcement and Appeals
  Guideline 8: Summary for Computer Bureaux
  Produced from the Office of the Data Protection Registrar, Wilmslow, Cheshire.

Fox, D.J. (1982) *Fundamentals of Research in Nursing*, Appleton-Century-Croft, Connecticut.

Hicks, C. (1990) *Research and Statistics: A practical introduction for nurses*, Prentice Hall, Hemel Hempstead.

Pollit, D. and Hunglar, B. (1983) *Nursing Research. Principles and Methods*, J.B. Lippincot, Philadelphia.

Treece, E.J. and Treece, J.W. (1986) *Elements of Research in Nursing*, 4th edn, C.V. Mosby, St. Louis.

5   The research process

The research process outlined

This chapter gives an overview of the research process. It is designed to be a source of reference rather than a definitive guide as to how to carry out research. Subsequent chapters will give more detail relating to some aspects mentioned in this chapter and cross-reference will be made to these as appropriate. Readers with specific research projects in mind are directed to the further reading section at the end of the chapter.

Defining the research problem

At the beginning of a research study there is a need to clarify the area of study and make a clear statement of what is seen as the research problem. Very often when reading research reports it may appear that the researchers have simply decided what they are going to study and begun their work in that area without any great difficulty. In reality, as noted in earlier chapters, most researchers start with a general idea of the problem area, which is subsequently refined to give a specific focus to the study. This refinement is achieved by a critical analysis of the subject area, based both on personal knowledge of the subject and on information obtained from the literature available. Quite frequently researchers will also have discussed their ideas in some depth with supervisors or colleagues to help to clarify their research ideas.

Following a period of consideration, discussion and a review of relevant literature the researcher should be in a position to clarify the area for research; that is, to define the problem area. This preparation time is seen to be a very important phase in the research process.

The literature search

As the next chapter explores this topic in some detail this section is included only to highlight some practical points about the literature search as related to

Table 5.1   Research process outlined

Defining the problem	
Searching the literature	Initial and ongoing
Designing the study	Clarifying the approach
The research method	Experimental, survey, case study, action research
Techniques	Questionnaire, interview, observation techinques
Population and samples	
Access	
Pilot study	
Collecting data	
Data analysis	
The research report	

the research process as a whole. The first point to make is not to underestimate the necessary expenditure of time required in searching for and reading the literature before beginning the actual study. This comprises quite a large part of any research project but is essential if the problem area of the research is to be clarified. The more knowledge that can be gathered in searching the literature the easier it is for the nurse researcher to identify which specific areas would benefit from further study. If the researcher has, for example, started thinking about research in a broad subject area such as communication in nursing she will find, in only a preliminary skim of available literature, that there is a need to reduce the area of interest to provide a specific focus for the research study. For example, she may decide to study a more clearly defined area such as communication in the health-care team. If this option was chosen the volume of available literature on the subject would be markedly reduced and consequently the nurse may be better able to clarify ideas for a research study.

Searching the literature can also help to indicate which approach to research would be most appropriate for the study. Information on the research methods utilised in studies undertaken into the subject area will help in this, for generally the strengths and weaknesses of research methodology are discussed in research reports.

Reading the literature also helps to avoid duplication or 'rediscovering the wheel'. Unless the researcher is aware of studies previously undertaken, she will not know whether or not what she has is an original piece of work. It may be a wasted effort to plan and implement a research study only to find at a later date that all the work has been done before and the evidence of that work is more than sufficient for the nurse's needs. The possibility of replicating research studies is another aspect that can be considered when reading literature.

Although one reason for searching the literature is to avoid duplication there is much to be said in favour of replicating reported research projects, particularly if they are small-scale projects. Factors such as sample size contribute towards the ability of the researcher in generalising the findings to a wide range of settings. The implications of small sample sizes are discussed in more detail later in this chapter, but it is worth emphasising that if a research study is undertaken with only a small sample it may not be possible to apply the findings in a variety of settings. This lack of ability to generalise findings can be a major problem to nurses looking for research on which to base their practices. As research is still a relatively new phenomenon in nursing many reported projects are still classed as small scale. The value of replication lies in the fact that if many small-scale research studies, exploring similar themes, were to result in similar findings then nurses can be more confident about utilising such findings in different settings.

It can be seen that literature searching can be used to clarify research ideas, to avoid duplication or to give the nurse researcher an opportunity to replicate a study.

Whatever the reason for undertaking a literature search it is essential to keep note of the source of reference material. This is a practical tip that is often overlooked when searching for information. Keeping accurate records which summarise reading is a good habit to get into for a variety of reasons. It certainly helps to avoid the frustration of being unable to relocate a piece of vital information that could be in any one of many books or journals. No doubt there are some people who have the capacity of instant recall, but unfortunately they are few and far between. For the majority it is advisable not to place too much reliance on memory when approaching a detailed literature search. Specific methods of keeping records are explained in Chapter 6.

Designing the study

Following a thorough review of the literature the researcher may find that some of the original ideas for the research project have been clarified or redirected. The problem area outlined at the beginning of the study may be modified or redefined, and clearly defined aims for the research project are identified.

Before a researcher can begin to collect data she needs to consider fully what approach she is going to take in her study. This ultimately depends on the overall purpose of the study and the questions the researcher wants to answer. If the nurse is seeking to predict outcomes as a result of her research study she will attempt to measure variables such as wound dressings and healing rate in an experimental study. However, if it was not possible for the nurse to utilise an experimental approach she may still seek ways of examining relationships by using a non-experimental, or descriptive, approach to research.

These approaches to research have come under close scrutiny in recent years as nurses have begun to question this scientific or 'positivist' view when undertaking research studies in nursing. Consequently, alternative approaches to research are being utilised; these will be discussed further in Chapter 7 while, for convenience, the focus in this chapter will remain on descriptive and experimental research.

Descriptive research

Descriptive research tends to make up a large part of the research available to nurses. Although the same principles of a scientific approach are applied to this type of research it is somewhat less complex than the experimental approach, in which the researcher may play a very active role in manipulating variables.

As the title implies, descriptive research seeks to describe what is happening in a given situation. The value of this approach is that it frequently opens our eyes to what is happening around us. Imagine, for example, the situation where a member of a ward team feels quite strongly that there is a shortfall of nurses working in that area and that to improve this situation it would be useful to present some facts to the manager of that unit. If the nurse were to undertake a small-scale study to determine how nursing time is used in that unit she may find that the results differ from expectations. She may, for example, find that nursing time is not used very well. If this is the case then there may be grounds for a change in practice on the basis of this descriptive study. Alternatively, the nurse researcher may note that although maximum efficiency is used in the deployment of staff there is still a shortfall in numbers of nurses available for the work required.

It may be useful to explore this example in relation to a specific aspect of care. In undertaking this study the nurse may realise that time is wasted in undertaking routine tasks that have been part of the traditional practices in the ward. Prior to the research study nobody had thought to question why certain activities were undertaken or, if they had, they had not followed the question with any objective line of enquiry. For example, many nurses have experienced the situation where the first task that was done in the ward area in the morning was the bed-making round. It is, of course, important for patient comfort and safety that their beds are made and kept clean while in hospital. However, if the nurse researcher were to find that in the mornings the nurses on duty spent about an hour of their time bed-making and then spent the rest of the time available to them rushing around complaining of lack of staff, she would be able to act on the findings of her small study straight away. The first option would be to consider a reorganisation of the ward 'routine' to ensure that, rather than maintaining the ritual of bed-making first thing in the morning, the nursing staff were deployed in giving direct care to patients. The bed-making could then be absorbed into the activities throughout the day, perhaps making better use of staff resources when there are quiet periods or an overlap of staff.

Alternatively, the nurse may feel that having demonstrated that the bed-making component takes a large part of the nurse's day but is an unavoidable part of that ward activity she would be in a stronger position to discuss alternative strategies with nursing management. She may, for example, be able to make a case for using bed-making teams in her ward or unit (a practice now adopted in some units). She may have been able to calculate that the work involved is that required by one full-time extra member of staff. Again, if good justification can be given this may be the way forward to increasing the staffing establishment, which was perhaps the object of the exercise in the first instance. If the nurse is able to present a well-researched problem to the administrators she will stand a much stronger chance of improving the situation than if she relies simply on rhetoric and emotional arguments and assumed knowledge based on traditional practice rather than fact.

One very important aspect of descriptive research is that it provides a baseline from which further studies can be developed. A researcher wishing to undertake a large-scale project incorporating experimental techniques must 'begin at the beginning'. For example, a nurse manager planning to undertake an experimental study to test the benefits of introducing new methods of organising nursing work within her unit may establish an experiment to test her ideas in two wards in her unit. She may proceed with her study and confidently conclude on the basis of her results that the organisation of work in Ward X was more beneficial in terms of deploying nurses than the method of organisation in Ward Z. If this nurse had failed to gather some descriptive data pertaining to the work-load in each area her work might be strongly challenged by staff on Ward Z on the basis that they cared for a different type of patient with very different needs to the patients on Ward X.

In summary, it can be seen that descriptive research has a value in exploring situations. In deploying a scientific approach to this type of research the nurse seeks to obtain objective information. The techniques used to gather data in descriptive research vary and will be examined in more detail in the next chapter.

Experimental research

Experimental research seeks to identify relationships between events. Unlike the situation in the school laboratory outlined in Chapter 1, in which chemical substances can be manipulated to identify a cause and effect relationship, in nursing research the subject matter is more commonly people and situations related to their health. This may be one reason why the experimental approach has not been as widely adopted as descriptive research. In manipulating situations in relation to people, controlling variables can be difficult and ethical dilemmas can arise.

The starting point for experimental research is the statement of a *hypothesis* which serves to clarify the direction of the study. A hypothesis is a way of proposing a relationship between two or more variables, or factors, being studied. In an experimental design the researcher has control over one of the variables stated in the hypothesis. This is known as the independent, or experimental variable. The second variable is known as the dependent variable. The hypothesis predicts that the independent variable will cause an effect on the dependent variable.

To facilitate statistical testing in experimental research it is normal to state a *null hypothesis*. In this statement a prediction of null effect, or no relationship between the variables, is made. Following statistical testing this statement may then be accepted as true or rejected as false. As an example to illustrate this approach we can take the situation in which a nurse believes she has found a cure for pressure sores. She may state her hypothesis that 'Treatment A results in the cure of pressure sores'. The null hypothesis would then be 'Pressure sores are not cured as a result of using Treatment A'. To test her hypothesis the nurse might select two groups of patients suffering from pressure sores. One of these groups would not receive Treatment A; this is the control group. The other group would receive Treatment A and is known as the experimental group.

This poses the first difficulty. In experimental research it is important that when two groups are studied they are similar in all the factors that may affect the outcome of the study. In this way any results found can be attributed to the effect of the treatment and not to the presence of one, or any combination, of these other factors. In ideal circumstances, therefore, this nurse would need to study patients of similar age, with similar health status and with similar pressure sore problems. It is not easy to find such similar sample groups. The second dilemma to be faced is an ethical one. If the nurse really believes that her treatment is best she is aware that in undertaking a study of this nature she is denying one group of people from a method of care she firmly believes in. This may cause anxiety to the newcomer to nursing research. What has to be remembered, however, is that this nurse has no evidence to prove that this new approach to pressure sore care is better than methods previously deployed. Her care to date has been based on intuition only and in the long-term interests of caring for her patients this experimental approach is necessary if research-based practice is to become fundamental to nursing practice. If the nurse feels that ethical dilemmas are likely to interfere with her ability to carry out a study she may need to consider alternative methods of testing the hypothesis. Exploration of the experimental method is beyond the scope of this book. The nurse interested in exploring this topic further should refer to the companion volume in this series (Hicks, 1990) which examines experimental research in nursing. In addition, readers are recommended to read published experimental research studies to determine specific strengths and weaknesses of this method as identified by individual researchers in their work.

Research techniques

The research techniques and design of research tools for collecting data are discussed in more detail in Chapter 7. The overall research design and aims of the study will contribute towards the decisions made about which techniques to deploy in data collection.

Population and samples

Access

In determining the population and sample size of the research study the researcher will need to consider how to gain access to the sample. Consequently, confidentiality and potential ethical dilemmas that might ensue should be addressed before seeking permission to undertake the study. As these issues have been discussed in the previous chapter the subject is included here only as a reminder that it should be considered as part of the research process.

Samples

Any nurse beginning a research study must consider the *population* and sample group that they will study. A population is a group of subjects having common characteristics. For example, all registered nurses may be seen as a population in a research study into nursing. A sample is seen as part of a whole. In research studies the population is the 'whole' that is to be studied while the sample selected for the study is seen as part of that whole.

The key factor to consider when determining both the population to be studied and the sample size is how far the researcher wishes to generalise her findings. If the findings of the study are to be widely generalised across the whole of nursing practice then the researcher must identify a *random sample* on which to base the research. This would represent a sample of a population with no bias factors in the selection process. The sample is said to be a true representation of a given population. This means that every member of the population being studied has an equal chance of being selected for the sample. For example, if the researcher wished to carry out an in-depth study of nurse training as a whole throughout the country she would need to ensure that all institutions responsible for training nurses were considered in the selection of the sample. This would be a mammoth task so she may attempt to become more specific in defining the population by excluding those groups undertaking degree programmes, as they represent a minority group with special needs. The remaining group is still large so a further exclusion may be done by making the focus of the study all those nurses who are training in large schools of nursing attached to a teaching hospital.

The researcher will still be left with a large population from which to select a sample for this study: the final sample selected may be done so at random. This could be achieved very simply by selecting names of potential participants out of a hat, or by making a decision to circulate questionnaires to every tenth nurse on the list of students obtained from the training institutions. Alternatively, the researcher may use one of several random sample tables available to researchers. Details and instructions on how to use these tables are generally included in texts on statistics. The references at the end of Chapter 8 can be used by readers wishing to explore random sampling further.

As the example above indicates, choosing a true random sample is possible but very unwieldy for many nurse researchers, even those who are full-time. Consequently, it is not uncommon for researchers to choose a *sample of convenience*. The researcher may decide that it is unrealistic in the time available to obtain a true random sample of student nurses in training throughout the country, so chooses to focus her study on a sample of convenience. For example, she may decide to focus on student groups in two or three large schools of nursing seen to be typical of schools of that type. In making this decision she may use fairly rigorous criteria to determine her choice of schools. In so doing she may, at the end of the study, be able to generalise her findings to some extent, but the limitations in sampling will be noted in the final report of the study.

If using a sample of convenience the researcher may still employ the principles of random sampling in determining which members of a given population will be studied. So, out of a group of 100 student nurses chosen as a sample of convenience for the study, the researcher may select a percentage of these, using random sampling techniques, as the final sample for the research. On a smaller scale a nurse undertaking a small research project as part of a post-basic nursing course may not have the time to identify a true random sample from a population of patients in the Intensive Care Units which are to be the focus of her study. Consequently, she will identify the patients in one or two local units as a sample of convenience. In making her report this nurse would not be able to assume that her findings relate to all patients undergoing intensive care but she may still identify factors that could be related to care at a local level.

It should be noted that although the results from such small-scale studies have only limited scope in terms of generalising findings to all situations, results from one small study might lend support to the findings of another similar study. Together these studies could be used to direct changes in practice if this were appropriate. For this reason there is value in replicating research studies in nursing.

Other factors affecting sampling

There are other issues that the researcher must consider when determining the sample for a study. *Organisational factors* may militate against the study of a given population; for example, a study may have been conceived which incorporates distribution of questionnaires to third-year student nurses in general hospital wards on a given day. It is quite feasible that the researcher's plan and the organisation's plan do not coincide for, on the chosen day, all third-year student nurses in that hospital are unavailable. Obviously, careful planning could help to avoid this situation happening but the example highlights the potential for changes within organisations to have an impact on a proposed study. A second point in relation to this is that *geographical factors* may also play a part in determining suitable samples. The nurse who decides to investigate the 'public image of nurses' may obtain totally different responses from a selection of people going in and out of hospital waiting areas to a random sample of people shopping in the main street on a Saturday afternoon. The implications are that this has introduced bias into the study. Awareness of the potential problem of introducing bias into a study is important. For example, if a nurse is undertaking a study of patients' reactions to their hospital experience she may find that a group of patients in hospital may give a different response to a group of people who have been discharged from hospital and had time to ponder on their experience. Both views must be considered in studies of this nature, as obviously location and potential vulnerability can make a difference to the way in which patients may respond.

Pilot study

The purpose of the pilot study is to identify any potential weaknesses in the design of the study. For example, if the method chosen to collect data is a questionnaire the researcher needs to know that respondents understand the questions asked and that the length of time taken to complete the questionnaire is acceptable. A pilot study is seen as a small-scale run of the major study and is therefore a useful exercise before embarking on the main project.

It is important that respondents in the pilot study reflect, as closely as possible, the sample of people that will comprise the population of the main study. Several factors will contribute towards the decision to undertake a pilot study. The first may be the research design itself; some methods of enquiry do not lend themselves to a 'trial run'. The size of the research project is another factor to consider. Some nurses may feel that there is little point in doing a pilot study if their proposed research is on a very small scale. For these nurses it is still advisable that some sort of *pre-test* is undertaken to test the validity of any research instruments used. A pre-test is not seen to be as complex as a pilot scheme but can produce useful information for refining research tools.

Following a pilot study the researcher may, if it seems necessary, modify the research tools before proceeding with the main study.

Collecting data

The methods deployed in collecting data are described by researchers in their reports. Any problems encountered are usually noted and the newcomer to research is advised to read these carefully, as recognition of the problems encountered by other researchers can help them to avoid similar problems. Further information on this aspect can be found in Chapter 7.

Data analysis

Research reports should carry clear accounts of how the results of the study were analysed. The researcher should consider how information, or data, collected should be analysed at the design stage of the research study. As with all aspects of research, careful planning in relation to this can help to avoid the pitfall of collecting copious information and not being too sure what to do with it once it has been obtained. In research reports the analysis of data should be clear, concise and reflect a fair picture of what was found during the course of the study. Methods of analysing and presenting data in descriptive studies are explored in Chapter 8.

The research report

The final part of any research study is the point where the researcher writes a full report of her work and findings. In concluding their work many researchers will make recommendations for action based on their findings. The reader of research reports should be alert to the style of presentation of information and make particular note as to whether the information in the final report matches the findings noted earlier in the study. In writing her report the researcher should obviously give an unbiased account of her study and her interpretation of the findings. As writing skills are seen to be a very important aspect of research this topic is discussed in more detail in Chapter 9.

Reading research reports

It is important that all nurses are able to read research reports in a critical manner. Obviously, the more critical the reader the better able they are to judge the quality of the research studies undertaken. This is an important point, for it must be acknowledged that not all research reported is good research and the newcomer to the subject must be alert to this fact. Because a research project has been reported in the nursing press does not mean that the findings should be adopted in every clinical area. Many factors contribute towards the quality of a good research project and nursing journals have differing criteria as to what is seen as acceptable material for publication. The nurse should clarify the status of the sources of information when reading and take care not to assume that all published research is good research.

To be able to read a report effectively the reader needs some insight into the research process. Consequently, it is felt that this chapter provides a useful source of reference for the nurse wishing to learn how to examine research reports critically.

Summary

This chapter has given an outline of the research process following the format noted in Table 5.1, and in highlighting the stages of the research process also gives a source of reference for nurses who wish to develop skills in analysing research reports. Insight into the stages of the research process and the potential problems faced by researchers provides a useful basis from which to review research literature.

Further reading

Calnan, J. (1984) *Coping with Research. The complete guide for beginners*, Heinemann Medical, London.
Calnan, J. (1976) *One way to do Research. The A–Z for those who must*, Redwood Burn Ltd, Trowbridge.
Cormack, D.F.S. (1984) *The Research Process in Nursing*, Blackwell Scientific, Oxford.

Darling, V.H. and Rogers, J. (1986) *Research for practicing nurses*, MacMillan Education, London.

Fox, D.J. (1982) *Fundamentals of Research in Nursing*, Appleton-Century-Croft, Connecticut.

Hawthorn, P. (1983) 'Principles of research: a checklist', *Nursing Times* (Occasional Paper), **29**(23).

Hicks, C. (1990) *Research and Statistics: A practical introduction for nurses*, Prentice Hall, Hemel Hempstead.

McCleod Clark, J. and Hockey, L. (1979) *Research for Nursing. A guide for the inquiring nurse*, HM & M Publishers, London.

Pollit, D. and Hunglar, B. (1983) *Nursing Research Principles and Methods*, J.B. Lippincot, Philadelphia.

Reid, N.J. and Boore, J.R.P. (1987) *Research Methods and Statistics in Health Care*, Edward Arnold, London.

Treece, E.J. and Treece, J.W. (1986) *Elements of Research in Nursing*, 4th edn, C.V. Mosby, St. Louis.

6 How to find information

What is a literature search?

Literature searching is a systematic method of accessing information. There is a vast amount of information published each year on nursing which can only be accessed effectively if a step-by-step approach is used. Techniques for literature searching vary according to the individual's needs, style and local circumstances but the basic approach and tools are the same. This chapter outlines the methods and gives explanations of the major bibliographic tools and searching techniques.

Libraries are a focal point for finding information and, like nursing and other health care professions, have their own subject language. You will therefore find words and terms in this chapter which will perhaps be unfamiliar or used in a different way. To help in understanding these, definitions are given of the major terms at the beginning of the relevant sections and at the end of this chapter in the Glossary. However, some of these terms are used differently from the definitions; for example, *Nursing Bibliography* is a Current Awareness Service which lists references in the same way as an index, mainly journal articles, and is therefore not strictly a bibliography.

The function of the literature search

The main functions of a literature search are as follows:

1. To ascertain and review the work already completed on a subject. This can provide contact with other researchers' work and prevent duplication.
2. To provide tools useful to the research project or clinical practice. For example: there are several scales used to measure pain. Only one may be suited to your particular purpose; a literature search will help to identify which one to use.
3. To provide support for research findings and/or their implementation. Other peoples' work is a valuable source of information on problems to help in validation of your own findings.

4. To validate results of particular tests or surveys. Test results may be peculiar to a particular environment; however, if research in other areas shows comparable results then a more general statement may be possible.

5. To help to define the extent of a research subject area. The first choice of research subject area may prove to be too broad, involving far more work than originally anticipated. As noted in Chapter 4, if starting with only a general subject area then the literature search can help to clarify ideas to produce a firm proposal.

Time

Literature searching can be extremely time-consuming but may ultimately save time in the practical stages of the research project. Allocating time to the literature search depends on environmental circumstances, such as library opening hours and the location of information sources. Approximately 10 per cent of the total investigation period should be allocated to the literature search. This can be divided into three elements, as follows:

1. A brief search to establish the extent of your proposal (1%).
2. A full literature search (6%).
3. A current awareness check throughout the investigation (3%).

Recording literature search results

A literature search may produce very few references or several hundred. Careful recording of references builds into an information-store on the investigation subject, avoiding the common problem of citing articles in the report and then discovering that the page numbers or journal issue number are missing for the reference listing. A good manual method of recording references is on a 5 × 3" index card – one per reference. The information on the card should be set out as illustrated in Figures 6.1 and 6.2.

Copyright (photocopying)

Many libraries have photocopiers available for public use making it easy to photocopy articles or sections from books for future reference. The Copyright, Designs and Patents Act 1988 permits the copying of only one article per journal issue. For a book, no more than 4,000 words (approximately equal to ten pages) as one continuous extract, 8,000 words as a series of extracts, each not more than 3,000 words, provided that the total copied does not exceed 10 per cent of the whole work. In both cases only one copy can be made. For

AUTHOR
    Article title:
    Journal title: volume; issue; date
    other identifiers e.g. 'Supplement'
    page nos.
    Source: (Bibliographic service, e.g. INI)*
    Location: (of journal, e.g. School of Nursing
        Library)
    Comments:

* If there is any problem obtaining the journal, this can help the librarian.

Figure 6.1   Index card reference for journal

AUTHOR/EDITOR – (Ed.)
    Title: (edition): place of publication:
    Publisher: year of publication.
    ISBN*
    Source: (Bibliographic service, or library
        catalogue)
    Location: (which library)
† Comments:

* The ISBN or International Standard Book Number is important if it is found necessary to purchase the book. It is unique to each edition of a title and therefore helps the bookseller to find exactly the edition required.
† The 'comments' section can be used for summaries and value to the research investigation. These cards can then be filed alphabetically and/or by subject.

Figure 6.2   Index card reference for book

Crown Copyright material – that published by HMSO, but also including the output of Government Departments and Government sponsored bodies – the terms are different. For a full explanation of these, refer to the *Library Association Record*, June 1986, 88(6), p. 286, or Her Majesty's Stationery Office, Copyright Section(P6), St Crispins, Duke Street, Norwich, NR3 1PD. Copyright law in the UK at the time of writing has just been amended. If in doubt, ask the librarian for advice.

Choosing a library

At the end of this chapter there is a list of major UK libraries which may be able to provide help and advice as well as printed information.

A great variety of libraries are involved in the dissemination of health-related information. Teaching districts, especially where there is a large medical or nursing school, are particularly well served. Levels of service offered range from a few books and journals to large stocks of academic libraries. Rights of access also vary considerably. Most non-nursing libraries will allow nurses at least a reference service and those which act as Regional centres will usually allow qualified nursing staff full access. Choosing a library therefore needs careful consideration. The main points are outlined below.

Access
Does the library allow nurses the full range of services?
Are opening times convenient to your off-duty hours?
Is a qualified librarian in attendance all the time and if not, on which days?

Stock
Is there a library guide or signposting for the stock?
Does the library have the main indexing and abstracting services for nursing literature?
Are most of the journals or books you are likely to require available in the library?
Is the library part of a loan/photocopying network and/or does it have access to the British Library photocopying and loan services?
Does the library have any special collections such as Official Publications or unpublished research reports?

Services
Is there a photocopier or photocopying service and how much does it cost?
Can you borrow a book?
Can you reserve a book out on loan?
How many books can you borrow and for how long?
Does it offer an on-line searching facility?

Environment
Is the library pleasant to work in?
Can it be easily reached from your place of work or your home?

Different libraries serve different needs and their style of service and stock will reflect this. Medical libraries will have large collections of journals, whereas nursing libraries will have a proportionately larger book stock. The Royal College of Nursing Library and the King's Fund Centre Library reflect two contrasting styles of service. The former is designed to allow maximum personal access to the stock by its members and presents a traditional library profile of open shelves of books. The latter is designed to deal mainly with written or telephone enquiries and therefore has a smaller book stock, almost entirely for reference, but an extensive collection of files on specific subjects. The *Library Association Directory of Medical Libraries in the British Isles* will assist you in finding a library in your local area. If this is not available to you, central public libraries may be able to help.

The literature search

Before starting the search it is important to establish the limits of the information needed. The following guidelines will help you to do this:

1. *Define your question.* The research proposal will have defined the intention but for the literature search a one-sentence definition that contains all the elements of the proposal is needed. The sentence should include subject keywords from which it is possible to search the library indexes and catalogues. An example of a poorly expressed sentence is: 'Facilities for relatives in intensive treatment units.' The words 'facilities' and 'relatives' are vague and liable to produce large numbers of references which have nothing to do with the actual question being asked. Be as precise as possible in formulating the sentence. A well-expressed sentence might be: 'The provision of family accommodation for intensive treatment unit patients in Britain.'

2. *List the synonyms of the keywords and terms.* This should allow for international variations in terminology and spelling as well as alternative indexing terms. Indexers use the main subject keywords of an article to produce the index subject headings; however, they will also limit the number of index headings under which an article can appear. Relevant articles may not, therefore, appear under the initial search term. In the above example it is possible to list the following.

Intensive Treatment Units (UK)
Intensive Care Units(USA)
Coronary Care Units (related heading)

Respiratory Care Units (related heading)
Critical Care (related heading)

Most indexing services include a subject headings list or thesaurus which will help to do this. The international variations must be included because, for example, the two major international nursing indexing services, *International Nursing Index* and *Cumulative Index of Nursing and Allied Health Literature*, are both produced in the USA and therefore reflect practice and philosophy in that country.

3.   *State geographical and language limitations.* For the example given, the interest is in British hospitals. Stating this will therefore help to limit the references found to those most relevant to the question. Care should be exercised, however, as comparative data can add validity to conclusions. Translation services are often expensive, so excluding non-English language material can save money.

4.   *Set a period to be covered by the search.* Information before a certain date may not be relevant. Retrospective coverage of five years for journals is a reasonable guide – the references at the end of articles will indicate the key older works.

When starting the search use the broadest subject term first. Many indexes will refer to related headings which can be explored after exhausting the main term. Make a note of any possible alternatives; they may contain references not obviously related to the subject but still of relevance.

Beginning the search

The literature search can begin with either books or journals depending on the subject and existing knowledge. Books provide a statement of established knowledge, whereas journals give the current state of knowledge, much of which will never appear in book form. Books also provide introductions to a subject and are therefore a good place to start if personal subject knowledge is limited.

The tools of the search

The tools of the search are those services available in the library giving access to the information required. Choosing which tools to use will depend upon which are available. Very few libraries will stock all, especially those for journals. Where there is a choice, evaluate each service according to the needs of the investigation; e.g., where a general clinical problem is being studied, *Index Medicus* may be a better choice than *International Nursing Index*. The services for books and journals are different.

Books

The library catalogue

The library catalogue is a complete listing of all the books in the library. The most common format for the catalogue is cards, but microfiche and computers are increasingly being used by larger libraries. Whichever the format, the information contained in each entry and the overall arrangement of the catalogue is the same.

Each entry will include, as a minimum:

Class mark

Author/editor (ed.)

Title; edition; place of publiation
publisher; year of publication

Library accession number(s)

These will then be arranged alphabetically by author's name for the Author Catalogue and by subject code for the Class Catalogue. The classification scheme used will differ between libraries but there will be a guide available in the library.

Bibliography

A bibliography is a list of books of any particular subject, author or country. Some libraries prepare bibliographies listing key material on particular subjects, including journal articles, serving as good introductions to a subject. Commercial bibliographies vary considerably in scope and comprehensiveness and should always be used with care. Check the scope notes – the publisher's introduction – before using them. Two commercially produced bibliographies may be of particular use:

1. The British National Bibliography (BNB)

This is a subject catalogue of all the British books received by the Copyright Receipt Office of the British Library. *BNB* is published weekly with four-monthly and annual cumulations since 1950 and thus forms a reasonably comprehensive listing of all the books on nursing and related subjects published in Britain.

Uses
To ensure that all the relevant titles published have been found.

Problems
Because of the cost only large libraries, such as central public or academic libraries, have publicly available copies.
It is time-consuming to check thoroughly.
Titles listed have not always been published.
Titles may not be easily available within financial and time constraints.

2. *The Bibliography of Nursing Literature.*

Details
Bibliography of Nursing Literature 1859–1960: with an historical introduction. Ed. by A.M.C. Thompson   London: Library Association; 1968.
Bibliography of Nursing Literature 1961–1970. Ed. by A.M.C. Thompson London: Library Association; 1974.
Bibliography of Nursing Literature 1971–1975. Ed. by Frances Walsh London: Library Association; 1985.
Bibliography of Nursing Literature 1976–1980. Ed. by Frances Walsh London: Library Association; 1986.

Uses
These four volumes form a useful overview of the literature of nursing, especially invaluable to anyone researching the history and development of the profession. They include journal articles as well as books.

Problems
They are limited by their nature to particular areas of research.
They are not comprehensive.
Availability of titles listed in the first volume may be a problem.

Directories
Directories can be useful sources of information. There are many organisations whose printed output is not listed anywhere and very often is not collected by libraries, but may still be relevant to the investigation. The types of material included here are help and advice leaflets, annual reports, booklets and research reports made available only from the organisation. Three particularly helpful directories which list organizations, their services and whether they publish follow:

Directory of British Associations (8th edn) ed. by G.P. Henderson and

S.P.A. Henderson   Beckenham: CBD Research; 1986.
Councils, Committees and Boards (6th edn) ed. by L. Sellar   Beckenham:
CBD Research; 1984.
The Mental Health Foundations' Someone to Talk to Directory ed. by D.
Thompson *et al.* London: Mental Health Foundation; 1985.

For the nurse needing information on other health authorities, such as names
and addresses, the *Hospital and Health Services Yearbook*, published by the
Institute of Health Service Administration, is a comprehensive listing of all
the Health Authorities in Great Britain.

Problem
Directories become dated quickly.

Sourcebooks

Sourcebooks can provide explanations and listings of, for example, organisations, legislation and information services. Two good examples are as follows:

Nursing and Midwifery Sourcebook Arnold Lancaster   London: George Allen
   and Unwin; 1979.
Health Studies: a guide to sources of information Audrey Cook *et al.* Newcastle upon Tyne: Newcastle upon Tyne Polytechnic Products; 1979.

Problems
Can become dated quickly.

Statistics

Sources of statistics can be divided into two categories, national and local.
National statistics can be found in the publications of a range of government
departments and organizations, such as the Department of Health, the Central
Statistical Office or the Office of Population Censuses and Surveys. Because
of the multitude of sources available, the Central Statistical Office produces an
invaluable guide:

Guide to Official Statistics Central Statistical Office, London, HMSO.

Local statistics can be very difficult to obtain. Some local government departments produce information on the demography of their area. Family Practitioner Committees produce annual reports as do Regional and Local Health
Authorities, but the statistical information contained in these is often very
broadly based. The information resulting from the implementation of the
reports produced by the Steering Group on Health Services Information

(chaired by Mrs. E. Korner) should be available from the District Information Departments, but may not be in a form which can be easily used. For example, admissions to an Accident and Emergency Department will be noted by diagnostic group, not by cause of injury.

Journals

Journals provide the most recent statements of knowledge on a subject. The vast number of journal titles published each year have meant that specialist support services have been created to provide systematic access to their contents. Two major types now exist, indexing and abstracting services, the difference being in their approach.

Indexing services (including citation indexes)

Indexing services list by subject and author the principle contents of selected journals. A basic entry will include the article title, author, journal title, date, volume number, issue number and page numbers. Citation indexes are a recent specialised form of indexing, based on the premise that references to an article give an indication of the article's importance, and provide a subject link between articles. They can also be used for tracing the development of a subject and for identifying the key authors, the 'authorities'. Citation indexes can be difficult to use effectively.

It is important for any indexing service that the publisher's statements on the criteria for selecting journals and articles are read. These will indicate the scope of the service and whether any types of material, such as government reports and theses, are excluded.

There are two major international indexes for nursing:

1.   International Nursing Index (INI)

Published by   American Journal of Nursing Company.

Frequency   Quarterly. The fourth issue is a cumulation of the year.

Arrangement   Alphabetically by subject and author. The subject headings follow the pattern of MeSH (*Me*dical *Sub*ject *H*eadings), which is the authoritative list of terms produced by the National Library of Medicine in the USA and used by *Index Medicus*.

Entries   Each entry includes: title of article, author, journal title, year, date, volume, issue and page numbers. Where the original is not in English, the entry is denoted in square brackets with a language designation at the end.

Other
services

Lists all the journals indexed. Annual cumulation includes a nursing thesaurus. Since 1986 a nursing citation index has been included in each issue. Annual cumulation includes lists of publications of organisations and agencies; nursing books published; dissertations (doctoral); and nursing-related data sources. None of these lists are comprehensive.

Positive
points

INI is easy to use.
Use of *MeSH* means that transferring a search to *Index Medicus* is reasonably simple.
MeSH is constantly updated, taking account of changes in subject knowledge and vocabulary.
Indexes all articles in each nursing journal issue.

Problems

As is common to all international indexing services, obtaining the source material can be a problem.
Authors sometimes use very abstract or cryptic titles for their articles.
There is no indication, other than the subject heading, of article content.
It does not give comprehensive coverage of British nursing journal titles and therefore should not form your only source of reference.

2. *Cumulative Index of Nursing and Allied Health Literature (CINAHL)*

Published by   CINAHL.

Frequency   Bimonthly with annual cumulations.

Arrangement   Alphabetically by subject and author. The subject headings follow a very similar pattern to *MeSH*, though they are produced by CINAHL.

Entries   Title, phrase from content (giving a qualifier for the title), author, descriptors, journal title, year, date, volume, issue, page numbers and number of references.

Other
services

Subject listing of new books.
Annual list of subject headings.

Annual list of book reviews.
Annual list of audio-visual materials.
Annual list of pamphlets.

Positive points	Easy to use. Use of qualifiers and descriptors means that relevance to your research is better judged. Books listing can act as a partial current awareness service.
Problems	Obtaining journals can be a problem. Search terms can only be used effectively with CINAHL. Does not give comprehensive coverage of British nursing journals.

There are many other indexing services which can be of use; for example, general medical subjects:

Index Medicus, produced by the National Library of Medicine in the USA and published monthly with annual cumulations, covers many of the journals included in *INI* but not as exhaustively. If *INI* and *CINAHL* are not available, then *Index Medicus* is a good alternative.

Or, for the social sciences, *British Humanities Index*, published quarterly, covers a wide range of social science subjects.

Many journals produce their own annual indexes, though these are not always of good quality.

Abstracting services

Abstracting services differ from indexing services in that they give a summary, or abstract, of the content of the entry. To be reliable the abstract should contain what the author has set out to achieve, the methods used to achieve the results and whether they have been achieved. The abstract should be signed, preferably not written by the author or journal editor and not less than one hundred words. Independent authorship of the abstract means that any problems of subjectivity will be reduced and the signature reveals authorship. One hundred words is the minimum needed to convey enough information to make a considered judgement on the usefulness of the item to the investigation. Careful use of abstracting services can save a great deal of time and expense in not having to check every possible reference, at source, for relevance. The major abstracting service designed for nurses in the UK is discussed below:

Nursing Research Abstracts (NRA)

Published by	The Department of Health and Social Security, Index of Nursing Research.
Frequency	Quarterly.
Arrangement	By subject with an author/subject index. The subject grouping of the abstracts covers very broad areas, such as 'Mental Health', so it is essential that you use the subject/author indexes. Subject terms are those used by the *DHSS Thesaurus of Health Care Terms* used in the DHSS Library.
Entries	Each entry gives the author, title, journal, date, volume, issue and page numbers. Books and theses are also included and their entries are different, though author and title are also used as the first entry components. The abstracts are of high quality and mainly produced by the DHSS staff. Where a journal or author abstract is used it is indicated. Ongoing and recently completed, but not yet published, research is also included.
Services	Annual author and subject indexes.
Positive points	Good quality abstracts. The expressive style of the indexes makes it easy to use.
Problems	Obtaining material is not always possible, especially for ongoing and unpublished research.

Other possibly useful abstracting services are *Health Service Abstracts, Hospital Abstracts* and *Quality Assurance Abstracts*, all produced by the DHSS. *Hospital Abstracts* has recently become part of Current Literature on Health Services – see page 61.

Current awareness services

One of the major problems of indexing and abstracting services, that of delay between journal and index publication, is partly overcome by current awareness services. A current awareness service endeavours to give coverage of a specific subject or group of journals for a specific reader group. Each entry gives the minimum information, usually arranged by subject, the service being published with the minimum delay from journal publication. Many libraries produce their own for specific groups within their area; for example, the West

Midlands Regional Health Authority Library's *Current Awareness Bulletin*, published fortnightly within the Region for senior managers. Current awareness services do not usually give comprehensive coverage of the contents of journals, simply the items of interest to their reader group. Many also offer a photocopy service for obtaining listed articles. Several nationally available health-related services exist, the Royal College of Nursings' *Nursing Bibliography* giving the best coverage for nurses in all disciplines.

Nursing Bibliography

Published by	The Royal College of Nursing.
Frequency	Monthly.
Arrangement	Alphabetically by subject.
Entries	Author, title, journal, issue, date and page numbers. When a title does not give a clear indication of content, extra descriptors are used.
Other services	Photocopy service. Annual list of subject headings. Annual list of journals indexed.
Uses	Can be used as an indexing service.
Positive points	All entries are available from the RCN Library, either by photocopy (journal articles), loan (books) or by personal visit (theses and reference only items).
Problems	Tendency to fall behind in its publication schedule.

Nationally available services also include *Current Literature on Health Services* and *Library Bulletin*, both from the DHSS Library, the latter for books added to the Library's collection. An unusual but highly effective current awareness service designed for midwives is *MIDIRS*. This service is published three times a year as an information pack, which is collected in a loose-leaf binder. Each pack includes reprints of journal articles, abstracts, reviews of new books and editorial comment. The last pack for each year includes a directory of voluntary and statutory organisations in the UK involved in maternity care. It can be used as a current awareness service, a directory and as a source of original material.

On-line (computer) retrieval systems

Availability

Although not yet widely available, on-line retrieval systems are an important tool for accessing the contents of journals. Access for nurses is limited to a very few centres, such as medical schools and some schools of nursing. However, the Royal College of Nursing and the King's Fund Centre undertake searches by request.

What is an 'on-line retrieval system'?

On-line retrieval systems are, in this context, indexing services made available electronically, for a fee, to anyone with a computer terminal connected to the telecommunications network and a password to a database host.

Development

The information explosion of the late 1950s and early 1960s, which saw a dramatic increase in the number of journal titles being published, meant that existing journal indexing services had to find alternative means of processing their information for publication. Moving from manual to electronic processing was the answer, allowing publishers to process and store greater volumes of information in a shorter period. Organisations such as the British Library soon realised that the computer tapes could also act as indexes in their own right, giving faster access to updated material than their printed counterparts. However, at this time processing a request and producing a reference listing took up to 14 days, faster than the printed indexes but not always as accurate.

The next step was to make several index databases available at one centre and, with the development of faster computers and operating systems, to make these available to remote users via the telephone network – on-line. DIALOG in the USA was the first centre – 'host' – in 1966. There are now many more giving access to several hundred databases around the world. Improvements in computer technology have meant that the databases are no longer simply electronic forms of printed equivalents but services in their own right, offering easier access through search strategies not possible to duplicate in print. There are also several databases which do not have a printed equivalent. On-line literature searching has several advantages over manual, but there are also disadvantages, some particular to nursing.

Advantages

Faster updating giving greater currency.

It is possible to search most databases using any term. The database does not rely on author or subject indexes, making it possible to search for terms and names as they appear in the entries.

By combining terms it is possible to have greater specificity and therefore higher levels of accuracy (relevance) of retrieved references.

Several databases can be searched from one physical location, far more than it is usually possible for a single library to provide in printed form.

Printed copies of the search saves on note-taking – recording references by hand.

All references can be seen together, not spread through several volumes.

The search intermediary – the librarian carrying out the search on your behalf – will be able to give advice prior to and during the search.

Most searches take less than 30 minutes.

Disadvantages

COST. This is the most important consideration when charges of £20–40 can be achieved for a single search. Costs can be broken down into (a) telecommunication charges, (b) a fee for using the host and each database and (c) a fee for each reference printed. (a) and (b) are calculated on the basis of time, so the longer the search takes the more it costs.

Obtaining source material is as much a problem as it is for printed indexes.

Few databases index nursing material.

Costs can be limited in several ways. Precise search strategies should be worked out, as for a manual search, before commencing – if one fails, have a second ready for immediate application. Check the database fees before starting the search – one database may be very much cheaper than another and will cover your subject just as well. The librarian who conducts the search will be able to advise on the choice of database and help to organise the search strategy.

Table 6.1 contains some of the databases which include nursing and health-related material.

Obtaining search results

This can be a problem. Theses and unpublished research papers present a particular problem as there is usually only a single copy available for public inspection. Many libraries will have a collection of locally produced material, while the Royal College of Nursing *Steinberg Collection* is a useful national source. Gaining access to the material may involve travelling to the holding library.

For books, most nursing libraries do not belong to inter-library loan networks, but public libraries do and will obtain titles if you supply all the bibliographic details.

With journals, the difficulty lies in finding a source library. If your local nursing library is part of an inter-library photocopy network then most of your

Table 6.1   List of some databases which include nursing and health-related material*

Title	Printed equivalent	Subject content
Nursing and allied health literature	CINAHL	Nursing
Medline	Index Medicus (including INI)	Medicine
Sociological abstracts	Sociological Abstracts	Social sciences
Psychological abstracts	Psychological Abstracts	Psychology and related disciplines
DHSS–DATA	DHSS indexing and abstracting services	Health service administration, management and nursing research
Cancerlit	None	Cancer: treatment, epidemiology, pathogenesis, immunology
BMA press cuttings	None	Summaries of articles and information in the media on health issues

* Not all host services will have all the above databases.

needs should be met. The library may also have access to the British Library Document Supply Centre (BLDSC) for journals not available locally. If neither of these services are available, libraries such as those at the King's Fund Centre, Royal College of Nursing and the Royal College of Midwifery will supply photocopies of articles upon personal application.

Fees must be charged by libraries for photocopies and this must be taken into account when selecting references, especially when only limited funding is available.

Writing references

If a written report is produced at the end of the investigation, the relevant results from the literature search should be included.

Why write references?

References are needed so that credit can be given to authors whose intellectual efforts have been used. They allow the reader to see from whom information was derived and give the opportunity to read further on a subject. They help in checking the validity of statements, whether quotations have been used in context or results interpreted accurately. They also give readers an opportunity to update their own information on the subject. References must therefore contain enough detail for readers to be able to find the source material.

Reference list or bibliography?

Reference lists and bibliographies serve two slightly different functions. Reference lists contain those items referred to directly in the text, either by quotation or author's name. A bibliography lists readings which are relevant to the work but have not been referred to directly. Inclusion of a bibliography is optional.

Connecting references to reference list

There are two popular styles of connecting references to the reference list; they are equally effective:

1. The Harvard system

This system is perhaps the easiest for the reader in that the reference list can be arranged alphabetically by author's surname and is therefore quick to check. The Harvard system links reference to list by giving the author(s) and date in the text, thus:

> Mumford (1986) lists the drugs commonly administered via a nebulizer as . . .

or, in the case of direct quotation:

> 'Jet nebulizers are used extensively on medical wards for the administration of drugs . . . ' (Mumford, 1986).

When two works by one author from the same year have been referred to, they can be differentiated by using, for example, (1986a) and (1986b). The reference list should be arranged alphabetically by author's surname and, when more than one work by an author, in chronological order.

2. Numeric or Vancouver system

This numbers references consecutively as they appear in the text or as they are arranged in the reference list. Using the above example the text would read:

Mumford[1] lists the drugs . . .

Journals
The full reference should contain the following details.

Harvard System
Mumford, S.P. (1986) Using jet nebulizers *Professional Nurse* Jan.
    Author   *Article title*   *Journal*   *Date*
                1(4), pp. 95–9.
                Vol. (Issue); Pages

Vancouver System
(1) Mumford, S.P. Using jet nebulizers *Professional Nurse* 1986 Jan.
    Author   *Article title*   *Journal*   *Date*
            1(4), pp. 95–9.
            Vol. (Issue); Pages

The journal title should be distinguished by using capitals, italics or bold print.

Books
The system for books has two variables, editor or author and edition. For a first edition it is not necessary to make an edition statement.

Harvard system
Tortora, G.J. and Anagnostakos, N.P. (1987) *Principles of anatomy*
        Author(s)/Editor (Ed.)   *Title*
and physiology (5th edn) New York: Harper & Row.
      (Edition)   *Place of*   *Publisher*
            publication

Vancouver system
(1) Tortora, G.J. and Anagnostakos, N.P. *Principles of anatomy and*
        Author(s)/Editor (Ed.)   *Title*
physiology (5th edn) New York: Harper & Row;   1987
     (Edition)   *Place of*   *Publisher*   *Year*
           publication

If there is an editor, give the editor's name(s) and put (ed.) before the title. Many publishers list several offices. Always give the place of publication as the one listed first, usually on the title page. If there are any other details, such as the chairman of a committee for a government report, this should be shown, in parentheses, at the end of the citation. Variations in the order of the above pattern will be seen, but the basic information contained in the citation does not vary.

Copyright registration of original material

Claiming copyright of original material is important. It provides legal protection of intellectual property – an author's original work – and ensures that credit is given when original work is used by another author. A record of the date of writing is the essential factor in ensuring that copyright is protected. To claim copyright of original material is a simple process achieved, for example, by any of the following methods.

Registered post
Sending a manuscript by registered post to yourself and not opening the envelope when it arrives will provide a record of the date. However, any sign of tampering with the envelope may invalidate this method if a legal action were to be brought.

Acceptance by a library
Many libraries will accept original manuscripts of research work and will record a receipt date in an accessions register – a list of all new material received by the library.

Acceptance by publishers
If a manuscript is accepted by a publisher the date of publication will serve as a copyright registration.

Ownership of copyright is not as simple. If the research and/or the writing of the manuscript is carried out at the behest of an employer, the employing organisation can claim partial or total ownership of the work. The same principle can also be used by funding bodies or organisations. Publishers also claim control of copyright when a work is published.

Summary

A literature search is time-consuming and can be very frustrating. It can also be an enjoyable exercise which will broaden knowledge of the investigated subject and provide tools to exploit in the information-gathering process of a project. This chapter has detailed a systematic approach to literature searching and explained some of the major services available to give access to the literature in the UK. As nursing research develops more services will become available and specialist services such as *Quality Assurance Abstracts* will become less exceptional. Use library staff as a resource; they have a good knowledge of literature search tools and how best to exploit them. If local services are not available, then make use of the national services, most of which can be used by telephone or letter.

Glossary

Listed below are some of the terms and abbreviations used in literature-searching resources.

pp.   Printed pages. Refers to pages without full page illustrations, etc. If illustrations are included, p. should be used.

et al.   *Et alia* – and others. Indicates multiple authorship.

Abstract   Precise summary of an article, report, etc.

Bibliography   List of books of a particular author, subject or country. By strict definition this term should only be used for books.

Catalogue   List of books held by one library.

Citation   Reference to a particular article, text, etc.

Index   List of references arranged systematically, usually by subject or author.

Reading list   Can be defined as the same as a bibliography, but includes journal articles. Used for works not cited in a text but of relevance.

Reference   Detailed information enabling a reader to find a book, article, etc.

Reference list   List of works cited.

Major UK libraries

This list only includes libraries that offer a service which is designed to meet the needs of Nurses, Midwives or Health Visitors. For the first three on the list, use of the full range of services is restricted to members. Non-members should always contact the Library service by telephone or letter before making a personal visit. The King's Fund Centre offer an information service best used by letter or telephone rather than personal visit.

Health Visitors Association
50 Southwark Street
London
SE1 1UN

Tel: 01 378 7255

Royal College of Nursing
20 Cavendish Square
London
W1M 0AB

Tel: 01 409 3333

Royal College of Midwives
15 Mansfield Street
London
W1M 0BE

Tel: 01 580 6523

King's Fund Centre
126 Albert Street
London
NW1 7NF

Tel: 01 267 6111

For specialist interests the *Directory of British Associations* indicates whether organisations have a library or information service.

7   Approaches to data collection

This chapter gives an outline of some of the methods and techniques used by researchers to gather data. Although some of the techniques described in this chapter can be used in experimental research these methods will not be explored further, as issues related to this have been discussed in Chapter 5.

Approaches to research

There are different schools of thought about approaches to research in nursing. At a very simple level of analysis one view is that the purpose of research is to gather data in an objective way for the purpose of prediction. This is referred to as the positivist, or scientific approach. The ethnographic perspective, in contrast, looks for meaning and understanding rather than measurable 'facts'.

In relation to this distinction the terms 'quantitative' and 'qualitative' research are now commonly used in nursing practice. The word quantitative implies some form of measurement and is generally used to describe research studies in which an attempt has been made to measure research data in numerical terms. Qualitative research takes a different approach in that the researcher looks for 'meaning'. Rather than being limited to a narrow range of responses in a questionnaire with quantifiable responses, for example, respondents may be asked to describe something in their own words. In analysing the information the researcher will be looking for meaning, or understanding, in the responses gained and will not attempt to categorise this in a numerical way.

Although experienced researchers may favour one option and follow that line of enquiry in their studies it may help the newcomer to research to note that there are advantages and disadvantages to both approaches. Because of this some research projects can be seen to have a mix of quantitative and qualitative approaches. Where appropriate this potential for mixing approaches will be highlighted in the discussion below. Ultimately, the research questions asked will help to indicate which approach to use in any research study.

Quantitative research

Quantitative research will be reviewed first, for this is an approach that has been used more commonly in nursing research. It has been fairly usual practice for the newcomer to research to plan to undertake a first study using quantitative research methods. This may be because this method is seen as easier in that the information, or data, gathered can be easily analysed and subsequently presented in a structured format. Alternatively, this may simply be due to the stage of development of research in nursing. As knowledge increases so more nurses are exploring alternative approaches to studying the world around them.

As the word quantitative implies, this approach to research utilises some form of measurement. A number of people can be asked to answer a series of questions in which the range of possible answers is limited. For example, respondents may be asked whether they agree or disagree with a statement made in a questionnaire. The number of responses in each category is totalled and the end result can be given in numerical terms.

The way in which a researcher may present data from a quantitative study is shown in Table 7.1. In this example the sample of people responding to the questionnaire totals 100. The researcher has noted that 45 respondents agreed with the statement, 39 disagreed, while the remaining 16 did not respond. The table also indicates the number of responses in terms of percentage ratings.

Many reported studies that have used quantitative methods of data collection utilise more complex statistical methods to analyse the results. Statistics are used to give additional meaning to research findings: statistical interpretation of data takes analysis of the information to a deeper level than simply listing the numerical response of using percentage ratings. However, the newcomer to research does not need to worry unduly about statistical analysis when first reading research reports. It is common practice for researchers to explain the meaning of any statistical interpretation in the research report. The next chapter will review issues related to analysing quantitative data in more detail.

Table 7.1   Recording quantitative data   *ch 4*

	Total	Agree	Disagree	No response
The number of respondents that agreed and disagreed to a question				
Responses	100	45	39	16
Percentage	100	45	39	16

Qualitative research

Although quantitative research is widely used there are many situations in nursing practice that cannot be satisfactorily studied in a way in which data is quantified. Consequently, there is an increasing interest in the approach to research which explores the subject from a different perspective, attempting to analyse the quality rather than the quantity of data collected.

The difference between quantitative and qualitative research can be illustrated by referring to the example given in Chapter 4, a proposed study to determine how people react to being told that they have a diagnosis of cancer.

If researchers planned to take a quantitative approach to such a study they might base their work on ideas from relevant literature and from their own experience in caring. They will therefore be starting their study with an assumed knowledge base. In this context they will describe any concepts or theories that they will be using and indicate how they are going to explore these issues. For example, after recognising that a diagnosis of cancer causes stress they will proceed to define what they mean by 'stress' and how it will be explored in the context of this study. They may do this, for example, by designing a stress 'scale' to measure individual responses to stress.

What the researcher is doing in this instance is taking a deductive approach to their work. That is, they are starting off with a general knowledge base of the subjects they are studying, stress and cancer, and attempting to apply it to a particular situation. The risk in this approach is that it will not really tell the researcher what it is they want to know. The depth of understanding of individual reaction will be constrained by the boundaries set in designing the study. Also, any information obtained is confined by the categories that have been predetermined by the researcher. The researcher may obtain answers to questions asked if they take this approach to their work, but insight into the real meaning to the individual of being told that they have cancer will still be limited.

Thus, one of the major drawbacks of research based on a quantitative design is the inability of the researcher to probe further and really to understand the reactions of the individual to a particular situation. Although trends can be identified in the group of people who have been diagnosed as having cancer a quantitative approach may be seen as inadequate in explaining how the population being studied have reacted to a diagnosis of cancer.

Consequently, qualitative research is an alternative method that can be utilised. This takes an inductive line of reasoning which works in an opposite direction from the deductive approach described above. Rather than testing preconceived ideas the researcher would seek to understand the issues from the point of view of the population being studied. Concepts and theories are generated from the respondents and emerge as the study progresses rather than the other way round.

In exploring issues from a qualitative perspective the researcher is not necessarily concerned with large samples and quantifiable data. They are concerned both with seeing things through the eyes of the respondents and with understanding the meaning of the situation from the point of view of the respondent. Research techniques used to gather data in qualitative research will vary. One method of data collection that may be used is the interview technique. Rather than using a structured questionnaire interview techniques in qualitative research will allow respondents to tell of their experiences or views *in their own words*. Researchers using this approach may describe conversations rather than a structured interview. Research that utilises interview techniques demands skill on the part of the researcher to ensure that no bias is introduced into the study. A good source of reference to the reader wishing to know more about interviews in qualitative research methods can be found in the text on this topic by Field and Morse (1985). The same authors note the complexity of analysing data that has been gathered in qualitative research. Following an interview, for example, in which a tape recorder may have been used to capture data, the researcher would have to derive some meaning from the information gathered.

Transcribing information from a conversational interview takes many hours. In addition, much skill in handling data is required to derive real meaning from this. Ultimately the researcher is seeking to identify themes or concepts that emerge from the data, but before they can do so all the information must be carefully examined and categorised with every effort made to avoid bias.

The presentation of information following a qualitative approach is in marked contrast to the quantitative approach. In the latter it is the researcher who has predetermined the categories of response and these are clearly defined from the outset. In qualitative research the themes reported have been derived from the research itself and have developed as the research progresses. Although the same principles apply when planning qualitative research, reports tend to be presented in a less 'structured' format than a quantitative study. When writing the report the researcher using qualitative methods will attempt to give the information in much the same way that it was presented to them by the respondents. In so doing categories of response are identified and explained by the researcher. A good example of this approach in nursing is the work undertaken by Melia (1982), describing student nurses' accounts of their experiences of being learners of nursing.

Themes, concepts or theories that emerge from a qualitative research study can subsequently be used to form the basis of a quantitative study if the researcher wishes to examine their ideas from another angle.

Mixed methods

It is not unknown for researchers to use a mix of both quantitative and qualitative methods when undertaking research studies. For example, a structured questionnaire may be used to obtain some quantitative data relevant to the study. This may be followed by a series of questions that are open-ended allowing the respondent to state, in their own words, their reactions to a given situation. If this mixed approach is well structured and the quantitative component of a study is complemented by a qualitative section the name given is *triangulation*.

Surveys

The purpose of a survey is to obtain information about a given population, and they are a popular means of undertaking research studies. Although there are different ways of carrying out surveys one of the most commonly used is the questionnaire. There is a degree of familiarity with the approach even for the newcomer to research. This may be because we are accustomed to using questionnaires in a variety of situations in everyday life; the use of questionnaires will be examined in more detail below (pages 78–9).

There are other ways of collecting information that can be classed as surveys although they may not involve direct contact with respondents. The researcher may seek access to sources of written information, such as medical records. For example in the hospital environment a survey may be undertaken of the medical records to assess the type of patients admitted during a twelve-month period. In common with other research techniques the researcher will still be working to a set of questions to structure the collection of information. For example, they may wish to know how many of the primagravida mothers admitted to a maternity unit in the past year were under 25 years of age. This information is available in medical records but the researcher may need to structure a research tool to allow them to collate information that may not necessarily be available in one section of the records. It is quite common in large-scale research studies to collect information from records and to collate this with data collected from other sources to give a comprehensive overview of a chosen research topic.

The ways in which information is gathered in a survey can vary. For example, the ideal way to study the reactions of a student group to their course of study would be to determine their reactions at the beginning of their course and at frequent intervals throughout, thus creating what can be seen as a *longitudinal* study. This, although an ideal, is a very difficult approach to research primarily because of the time commitment involved. Consequently, it is more common for the researcher to undertake a *cross-sectional* study which seeks to compromise this idealistic approach by obtaining a representative sample. Thus, in a study of student nurses in training, the researcher may not have three years to spend on studying the student population but would be able to choose a representative sample from a group of first-year, second-year and third-year students. The cross-sectional approach does have an advantage in that it enables the collection of normative data against which individuals can be compared.

Case study

The term 'case study' will be familiar to most nurses in that it has long been a common practice in nursing for students at both a basic and post-basic level to undertake an in-depth study of one patient as part of their learning process. These in-depth studies of nursing care can be seen as having similar aspects to those of a research-based case study. This approach to research is frequently referred to as being on the opposite end of the spectrum from that of the survey approach. Surveys rely on an approach in which a large number of 'cases' are studied and a consensus view drawn from the results. The case study focuses one situation, or a limited number of people within a common situation such as the workplace, who are studied in depth in an attempt to give meaning and additional insight into the subject under review.

In undertaking this in-depth analysis of a single situation the researcher can utilise a variety of techniques of gathering information to obtain a more complete picture. Information is gathered over a period of time, therefore the research is put into the context of factors in the past and present rather than focusing on the here and now, which is a feature of survey research.

It is acknowledged that the case study approach only gives a limited amount of information and so the ability to generalise findings is severely curtailed. However, the value of this method is that in focusing on issues that are really meaningful to one individual this type of study can serve to increase knowledge.

An increase in knowledge of this nature may lead people to examine their own situation more carefully, an aspect that is beneficial to nursing. The emphasis on 'why' rather than 'what' in this type of research makes the case study approach the preferred option for many researchers.

Advantages of case studies

Case studies in nursing research can be useful for they are well-suited to exploring many situations that provide a focus in nursing. For example, the progress of a student nurse could be studied through her training. Alternatively, an in-depth study of one patient undergoing a new treatment regime will give insight into the individual's need and reactions. In providing this information the researcher may be able to give indicators for future care of similar cases.

This approach to research also allows freedom in terms of the techniques that can be used to study the case. Observational techniques may be used but in addition the researcher may use interviews or questionnaires when exploring the network of contacts related to the individual case. For example, the researcher studying a student nurse as she progresses through her educational programme may wish to add the views of family and friends and colleagues to the study to give a more complete picture. Another advantage in the case study approach is that the researcher can define the boundaries of when to begin and end data collection. Rather than studying one student over a number of years the researcher might set the boundaries at one year of training only.

The findings from a case study can lead to action if, for example, factors that effect an individual are identified and the response in a similar situation anticipated. This benefit can be important in nursing care.

Finally, the wealth of information gained in a case study can generate ideas for future studies. New concepts and theories for testing can be generated, unlike some other forms of research when existing theories are tested.

Disadvantages of case studies

The major disadvantage of case studies is the lack of flexibility: findings cannot be generalised to a variety of settings. In addition, data gathered from one case study may be in conflict with that gathered from another because of individual variations. This might happen if the researcher undertaking a case study of a student nurse decided to examine more than one case, for example. Further disadvantages are related to the complexities of the research design. The researcher may have to decide whether to study many aspects of the individual case superficially, or a few aspects in depth. The wealth of knowledge that can be gathered in relation to any one case is enormous and can increase as the study progresses. Consequently, there is a need to determine the boundaries of the study. There is also a need to question whether close liaison with the researcher and subject introduces subjectivity to the study. Those people being studied may behave differently as a result of being observed. Subsequently the research report may be biased, an aspect that researchers must take every care to avoid.

A final disadvantage of this method is that the costs of this type of research can be large compared with other approaches.

Techniques of data collection

Researchers using the case study approach may use a variety of techniques.

For example, a researcher reviewing the effects of a nurse education programme may choose the survey approach to study the overall reactions of a group of nurse students to their course. To complement this work the researcher may then choose one student on whom to make an in-depth case study by monitoring all their experiences and reactions to the course. In-depth interviews may be used and, if relevant, observation techniques deployed in an attempt to study the situation in depth through the eyes of one student. Alternatively, in a clinical situation, a nurse may choose to study one patient undergoing one particular form of treatment in an attempt to identify the problems that people may experience when put in the position of being a patient. In addition to the information obtained from the case being studied information can be gathered from a variety of other sources; for example, an individual family, friends and work colleagues can be approached to participate. Therefore, data can be collected by using records, interviews, questionnaires and observation techniques.

Action research

The focus of action research is on specific issues or problems identified in a local situation. An action plan is developed to introduce change to resolve the problems identified, and subsequently the results are evaluated. Those people within the locality are involved in the research and because of this participation action research is seen as collaborative. As the work is evaluated as it progresses action research can be described as cyclical in nature. The problem-solving processes of assessment, planning, implementation and evaluation can be applied to this type of research.

At the assessment stage the specific problem would be identified. The researcher would plan a strategy to help solve that problem. In implementing the action plan she would begin to monitor the effects of the plan. Finally, the whole process would be evaluated and the views of all participants incorporated into the evaluation. This evaluation would then form the basis of re-assessment as the whole process, or cycle, begins again with any modifications necessary being made.

The action research approach is well utilised in nursing education where ongoing evaluation of courses results in changes and modifications based on student and teacher evaluation. This reflects the fairly well-developed use of action research in education as identified by Cohen and Mannion (1980). An example of this approach in nursing studies is provided by Lathlean and Farnish (1984), who undertook a project of ward sister training.

In utilising this approach the researcher needs to consider wide-ranging issues. As with all research studies the overall aim of the research will help to determine if this method is appropriate. The same point applies to the techniques utilised to collect data when evaluating the effects of the action. The advantage of using this approach is that it offers a means of solving local problems. Emphasis on introducing and monitoring the effects of a change in the environment can help to promote an interest in research among people who perhaps have not been involved in research studies before. Group participation also helps to motivate and maintain interest in the research which may be seen to be meaningful to participants, as the results of changes made can be monitored closely at the point of action. This is unlike other research methods in which there is commonly a time lapse between completion of a research study and implementation of a preferred action plan based on the findings.

The main disadvantage of using this method is that the findings cannot be generalised beyond the situation being examined.

Techniques used in data collection

The first section will focus on the use of questionnaires, including interviews and self-administered questionnaires. This will be followed by a review of observation techniques in nursing research.

Questionnaires

The aim of the research will determine how information gathered by questionnaires will be utilised. For example, if a number of student nurses were asked to respond to a questionnaire about their course of training the analysis may result in a simple descriptive study. In this there is no attempt to analyse the results beyond describing the information given. The researcher may, however, use the information gained in a questionnaire survey to analyse responses in more detail. This method may be used by researchers who, for ethical reasons, are unable to manipulate the variables in a study. For example, an ideal way to study the effects of nurse training schemes would be to introduce some control into the experiences available to the student group. By doing this the researcher would seek to identify both independent and dependent variables and to manipulate the situation to identify cause and effect factors. If they were to do this they would be undertaking experimental research. However, because of the constraints placed on nurse education it is not easy to establish such a clearly defined experiment. Consequently, if using questionnaires in a survey to study this topic the researcher could do a comparative study. Two groups of student nurses undergoing training in two different institutions could be asked to respond to a questionnaire. Although there has not been any control of the variables involved in the nurse education of these two groups, information gathered could still be usefully compared for any noticeable differences.

If information is gathered following a specific experience it is described as a retrospective study. The group of student nurses could be approached one year after completion of their course and asked to give their views of their training at that point. After a year of practising as qualified nurses their views may differ from those given on completion of their course. By this stage they will be in a better position to determine whether their training did indeed prepare them for their subsequent role as a qualified nurse. This approach has been used for evaluative purposes to determine the perceived value of the course on completion.

The use of questionnaires allows the researcher to gather facts or opinions related to a given topic. In gathering opinions surveys are seen as a good medium for measuring attitudes, motivation or values of respondents. In addition they are frequently used to predict events. For example, one form of prediction that we are all familiar with is that of predicting the outcome of general elections. The avid news-watcher at general election time will not only be used to hearing what the trends are in terms of public attitudes towards particular political parties but will have noted that the reporting of these has become rather more sophisticated as public awareness of research methods used has increased. Now news reports carry not only the results of various attitude surveys but proceed to describe the sample size and location of the study.

In nursing research the use of questionnaires to undertake a study has been very popular. The advantages of undertaking this approach do, to some extent, explain why this method is favoured, and are outlined in more detail below. At this stage, however, it is worth introducing a note of caution. Newcomers to research often think that it is easy to undertake a quick research study by producing a questionnaire and circulating this to their sample group. What they realise very quickly is that, however good the idea, it is actually very difficult to produce a good questionnaire. It is a useful exercise for all those nurses interested in research to attempt to design a questionnaire. The difficulties of doing this will soon become apparent and the level of skill required noted. In research terms a questionnaire is not simply a set of questions randomly put together; rather, it is a tool designed to explore specific research questions. Consequently, issues related to questionnaire design are discussed further in the chapter.

Methods of completing questionnaires

Interview techniques

Questionnaires can be completed by researchers meeting the respondents face to face and carrying out an interview. This method, although time-consuming, does have some positive advantages. In the first instance it avoids the problem noted below of the limitation of using self-administered questionnaires for those members of the population who are not literate or numerate. Respondents would not be faced with the embarrassment of explaining that they were not able to understand the questions asked in written form. Secondly, this method allows the researcher to ensure that forms are completed correctly; if not they have only themselves to blame. In addition, by completing the questionnaires themselves, the researcher is on hand to make any points of clarification required by the respondent.

Research interviews can vary in structure from a highly structured approach to one which utilises a more open approach. At one end of the scale of interview techniques the researcher using this approach would take a structured questionnaire and simply ask the questions as written and note the appropriate response. The interview is thus seen to be highly structured and provides a means of carrying out a *quantitative* approach to a research study.

At the opposite end of the scale from this highly structured format the researcher may take a more informal approach and ask open-ended questions that appear more general in nature and which allow the respondent more scope in their reply. Researchers using this technique will sometimes describe a conversational approach to this type of research interview. Information can be collected by writing down verbatim what the respondents say. Alternatively, tape recorders or video cameras can be used to capture information that is later transcribed for analysis. This reflects a *qualitative* approach to research.

The researcher using interview techniques to gather data will usually have undergone fairly thorough preparation before using this approach to ensure that they themselves do not introduce any bias into the proceedings. The researcher should be rigorous about keeping their own views out of the interview situation. To ensure that such objectivity is achieved it is often part of the research plan for researchers to undertake a period of training in interview techniques before collecting data in this way. If more than one researcher is involved in collecting the data, as happens in larger-scale studies, all those involved in gathering information will undergo preparation to ensure consistency in approach to their interviews.

Self-administered questionnaires

As self-administered questionnaires are a very popular means of collecting research data, particularly among newcomers to research, it will be useful to explore both the advantages and disadvantages of using this technique.

Advantages

The use of self-administered questionnaires allows the researcher to reach numerous people very quickly. It takes but a matter of minutes to circulate a handful of questionnaires to a sample of respondents. In contrast, interview techniques may take many hours, or even days, to acquire the same range of information from the same number of respondents. From this perspective it is easy to see why individual researchers may favour this method as it is feasible, in terms of time and effort, that one person could undertake quite a large-scale survey on their own. Another advantage is that the postal services can be used to reach a larger sample. Thus, for example, the nurse researcher undertaking a study of trained nurses could circulate questionnaires to a sample of 100 nurses in several health districts quite easily. Alternatively, if undertaking a study of patient satisfaction, it would be relatively easy to circulate 100 questionnaires to patients who have been discharged from hospital. It would be unrealistic for similar sample sizes to be obtained by the individual researcher using interview techniques if time was a major constraint in a research study. This is an important point, for the larger the sample for the research study the more likely it is that the researcher will be able to generalise findings.

Depending on the design of the questionnaire the results can be analysed easily. As will be seen in the section on questionnaire design below, closed questions are easier to analyse than open questions. Also, it takes less time for respondents to complete a questionnaire with closed responses, which is a factor that has a direct effect on compliance among respondents. A further advantage often credited to the use of self-administered questionnaires is that the format offers respondents anonymity, which in turn may generate objectivity in responses given. In replying to an anonymous questionnaire the respondent may be more likely to give an honest answer if he/she is confident that no one will know who has made that particular response. This is particularly so if the subject of the research study is a sensitive one.

These are some of the positive aspects related to the use of self-administered questionnaires as a research technique. As with all things, however, there are two sides to the story and some of the disadvantages may well outweigh the advantages in determining the research method used.

Disadvantages

Although the information so far has seemed to be in favour of utilising a self-administered questionnaire in research there are several major disadvantages that may be sufficient to persuade the researcher to seek an alternative approach. The first problem is that questionnaires are difficult to design. A poorly designed questionnaire will yield only poor results. It is important to note that it is difficult to write questions that do not introduce the risk of bias into the study. For example, the nurse wishing to ask patients about their views of treatment in hospital will find it quite difficult to formulate objective, un-emotive questions in relation to the emotive experience that the patient has undergone. It is not impossible to do so, but it is not easy to write unbiased questions in relation to some aspects of nursing care. Consequently it is worth re-emphasising that any nurse planning to undertake a research study will be well advised to seek help and guidance from someone who has already had experience of doing research and can act in the capacity of supervisor or mentor. The experienced, objective eye on a newly designed questionnaire can do much in helping to avoid the pitfall noted above by advising on any obvious error or bias before the questionnaire is used. In addition, as noted in Chapter 5, it is advisable to test questionnaires before use in the major study. A pre-test or pilot study will help to determine whether the questionnaire is interpreted objectively by respondents.

The risk of non-compliance by respondents is another disadvantage of self-administered questionnaires. This can be a major source of frustration for researchers who need to consider ways in which this problem can be kept to a minimum. To ensure optimum return rate the researcher must consider ways of distributing the questionnaires. Compliance can be linked to the fact that if left to complete questionnaires in their own time respondents may simply forget to do so. It is generally acknowledged that the method of posting questionnaires is likely to result in a lower return rate than those systems which allow the researcher direct contact with the respondents. If using postal services a 50–60 per cent response rate is generally seen as good, although this of course depends on the sample size and the nature of the survey. If this level of return is not achieved there are some strategies that can be used to increase the return rate. The inclusion of stamped addressed envelopes for return of the questionnaires is a useful tactic to reduce non-compliance. Another is to send out reminder letters to respondents if questionnaires are not returned. This frequently results in an increase in the return rate, but it does so at the cost of extra time and effort for the researcher.

An alternative approach, and one likely to yield better results, is to circulate questionnaires in a group setting if that is possible. This method may yield a response rate of 75–80 per cent (or higher) and this is seen as a good level at which to aim.

It is in the researcher's interest to consider alternative strategies for distributing questionnaires. For example, if wishing to carry out a survey of a 100 student nurses it may be helpful if they could be seen by the researcher in a group setting. This could, perhaps, be arranged if the group was attending a study day in the school of nursing as part of their course, which would allow the researcher to deliver and collect questionnaires personally, an aspect that usually ensures a high level of compliance.

Using these basic ideas the researcher studying a group of hospital in-patients could deliver the patient questionnaire personally to a sample of patients in hospital wards. There are implications in terms of organisation and timing for the researcher but the benefits of taking this approach in terms of response rate generally makes the effort worth while.

There are ethical issues associated with compliance in completing questionnaires. The offer of a reward, however small, affects the willingness with which people will complete them. In the business world large companies undertaking research have discovered this and may, for example, offer a reward such as a gift token as a sign of appreciation for participating in a study. It is recognised that human nature is such that offer of a reward or 'bribe' will have a positive impact on compliance. The researcher in health care does not have the option to offer bribes but this aspect should not go unnoted, for the principle can be applied in some areas of research. A sample of hospital patients asked to participate in a study while they themselves are in a vulnerable position may see refusal to participate in a research study as a factor that may affect the quality of care that they receive while in hospital. The researcher may know perfectly well that a refusal would be acceptable, but it is essential to remember that they are approaching this from a position of control, unlike the patient, who is in a vulnerable position and may not have insight into the health care system.

Equally, it may be thought that staff asked to paticipate in a research study have a choice. The staff may not see it that way if the person undertaking the research is a senior member of nursing management. It can be seen, therefore, that potential problems such as these should be identified at the outset so that no undue distress is caused to people asked to participate in research studies.

One further aspect that should be considered in relation to noncompliance is that some members of the sample group choosing not to respond to the survey may not have done so randomly. For example, if a midwife researching smoking habits in pregnancy was circulating questionnaires to pregnant mothers she may be very pleased to discover that the responses indicate a general reaction against cigarette smoking. However, further analysis of the questionnaire might reveal that all the respondents were non-smokers. The pregnant mothers who smoke may have chosen not to respond to the questionnaire and consequently their views are not represented in the analysis. This aspect of non-compliance can result in a biased result.

Another disadvantage of self-administered questionnaires are that they are only suitable for the literate and numerate. This may sound a fairly obvious statement but it is an aspect that can easily be overlooked. If we apply this point to a study of nurses and patients the problem can be illustrated further. The researcher may circulate questionnaires to nurses with confidence knowing that they will be able to complete the questionnaire. However, it is the level of literacy in a population over which there is little control or knowledge that may cause difficulties in using this technique. For a number of reasons, including dyslexia, inability to read or write English or simply poor educational opportunity, this sample may be unable to co-operate with a questionnaire approach. Consequently, the researcher should use this method with caution and take every care not to cause embarrassment.

Issues related to correct completion of questionnaires should also be considered by the researcher considering potential disadvantages of the approach. Accuracy in response is not possible to check. The design of the questionnaire and pre-testing before use will help to identify any weakness in the research design that may contribute to this, but the researcher has no control over the way in which respondents ultimately choose to answer. It is hard to deal with ambiguity and if a respondent does not make their meaning clear the researcher is not in a position to put their own interpretation on the response. It is not uncommon to read in research reports that a number of responses have not been used in the final analysis because they were 'spoiled', with the result that the response was not clear to the researcher.

One further aspect that should be considered in the research design is that there is a tendency in some people when faced with a questionnaire to look for the 'right' answer. This may be a result of schooling and habits of a lifetime. Alternatively, it may occur because the respondent wants to 'help' the researcher by giving what they see as the expected response. Again, a good research design should help avoid this pitfall.

Designing a questionnaire

Some of the key points that should be considered when designing a questionnaire are outlined below. This is not intended to be a definitive guide; rather, it is included simply to increase awareness of the kind of issues that must be considered when using questionnaires in a research study.

It is most important that the initial presentation is such that the respondent will not be immediately put off completing the questionnaire. The questionnaire design should match the interests of the group of respondents it is designed for. A good guide in this would be to consider the difference between picking up a large print, easy-to-read book and one which is in tiny print and has very cramped pages. The former would be more appealing to the majority of people looking for a 'light read' while the latter would perhaps appeal to the academic interested in the particular subject matter under review. For both groups, however, it is important to make the questionnaire presentable, easy to read and understand and easy to respond to.

Respondents should be advised about the *purpose* of the study. If questionnaires are to be administered in a group setting it is easy for the researcher to give this information verbally. Failing that, some form of written explanation must be given. This can be done at the top of the questionnaire. Alternatively, a short letter can be written to research subjects explaining the purpose of the study, requesting co-operation and giving any relevant instructions relating to completion and the return of the questionnaire. A guarantee of *anonymity* is important to ensure that respondents know that confidentiality will be maintained. It is also courteous to thank respondents for participating in the study indicating, if possible, how, when and where the results of the study will be available to them.

The *layout* of the questionnaire is important. As this has the first impact on the respondent it can serve to inspire interest and thus motivate co-operation. At the top of the page the researcher should indicate how they want the respondents to complete the questionnaire, giving clear and unambiguous *instructions*. The *amount of information* required on the front sheet of the questionnaire should be considered. It is a common practice, although not a rigid rule, to include any necessary *biographical detail* at the beginning of a questionnaire. Questions such as age, sex and place of work are usually addressed at this point, if they are relevant. Researchers must consider very carefully what additional information is included in this section and they should take care to ensure that only essential data is requested from respondents. Failure to do this may contribute towards non-compliance, as respondents can be very easily put off completing questionnaires if they think that questions are not related to the topic under review. For example, respondents may start filling out a questionnaire about their attitudes to work but, if faced with a question pertaining to a very personal aspect of their own life, may question the purpose of the study and stop their response because of this. They may suspect some ulterior motive behind irrelevant questions and, perhaps, question the integrity of the research.

Writing questions for use in a questionnaire research is an important issue. Questions that require a 'yes' or 'no' response or an indication of attitude to a given statement can be described as *closed questions*. The respondents only have a limited choice in the range of answers available to them but can still express a fact or belief in relation to the question asked. For example, a survey of the general public may be seeking to identify how many people are television owners. The question 'Do you own a television set?' will demand a 'yes' or 'no' response.

A variation of the closed question approach seen in some studies is the *'forced choice'*. The respondent is expected to make one of a number of choices from predetermined categories. This method does have some uses but can also be seen to be too limiting for some studies. This method could be used to determine if the respondent watches television once a day, once a month, once a year or never. In being forced to make a choice from one of these categories the respondent who watches television on a more erratic basis may be frustrated in trying to determine which of these responses fits their pattern of television watching.

Ranking scales are another example of recording responses in questionnaires. The respondent may be asked to indicate their strength of feeling on a given subject by selecting a point on a scale representing the poles of a continuum. In this way, the television watcher may be asked to indicate, on a scale of 1 to 10, in which 1 represents total enjoyment of television watching and 10 represents no enjoyment, how much they enjoy watching television.

All the approaches outlined above represent methods which would facilitate *quantitative research*. The researcher will be able to measure in numerical terms how the respondents reacted to a given question.

An alternative approach that may be used is to present *open questions*. The possible range of information gathered is increased. Depending on the research questions asked the data produced may be *qualitative* in nature if the respondent is given the opportunity to state in their own words exactly what they feel about a situation. Although open questions are frequently used and can generate much useful information for the researcher it is considerably more difficult to handle the information obtained. Each statement made by individual respondents will require in-depth analysis and consequently is more time-consuming than counting the number of positive or negative responses generated by a closed question approach. In utilising open and closed questions some research studies incorporate both quantitative and qualitative components in questionnaires. This mix of quantitative and qualitative methods is quite a useful approach to take to research for it allows more in-depth information gathering in relation to questions asked. In the final analysis the researcher will have quantitative information on which to base part of the report and this information can then be elaborated on by qualitative information available.

Regardless of the method of analysis the phrasing of the questions is important; thus, the writing of the questions is the most important aspect in preparation. They should be clearly written and unambiguous and should relate to the stated aims of the research. There should be nothing within the structure of the question that will lead to a biased response. The researcher should avoid confusing the respondents by including questions that include negative statements, or worse, double negatives. For example, if the respondent was asked to answer 'yes' or 'no' to the following statement they might be rather confused.

'If you do not turn the patient you are not giving good care.'

This is not a good question, because it is not clear to the respondent whether they are responding to the issue of turning a patient or giving care.

A better way of phrasing this would be:

'Turning a patient is essential when giving good care.'

It is a useful exercise for all newcomers to research to practice writing questions.

It is worth noting that the easier it is for a respondent to complete a questionnaire, the easier it is for the researcher to analyse the results. For example, if a questionnaire has a number of closed questions requiring simply a 'yes' or 'no' answer all the researcher has to do is to count the number of people who answered 'yes', compare this with the number who said 'no' and present the results. Equally, if the option is given for the respondents to reply to a number of statements which seek to identify attitudes by asking them to agree or disagree with the statements made, again there is a limited number of responses for the researcher to work with and the results are easily collated.

In determining the style of question and the method of response the researcher should also be considering how the data obtained is to be analysed. The newcomer to research frequently falls into the trap of setting a number of questions and not considering what will be done with the responses once they have been acquired. Advice from a supervisor in the early stages of a research project will help to avoid pitfalls that occur from the failure to forward plan.

There are other variations of questionnaire design open to the nurse researcher, but to introduce them here would only add to the complexity of the book. The further reading section at the end of the chapter provides a source of reference for the reader wishing to explore this further.

Observation techniques in nursing research

The overall aims of the research study will help the nurse to determine if she wishes to use observation techniques as a means of gathering data. Observation techniques can be utilised in both quantitative and qualitative research. If the researcher is looking for answers to specific questions they may choose to use observation techniques in a very structured way in which categories have been predetermined by the researcher. This form of observation may result in findings that can be measured and quantified. For example, as part of a study to measure nursing work-load the researcher may observe how many temperatures are taken in a ward area over a span of eight hours. Simply by placing a tick on the check-list each time a temperature is recorded, data is collected in an objective quantifiable way.

At the other extreme the researcher may choose to participate in activities in the area being observed. Rather than using an objective check-list their experiences are noted more informally, perhaps in diary form. Notes gathered in this way are commonly referred to as field notes, as data is collected from observing the subjects in their normal role of activity rather than in a more controlled environment such as a laboratory. In giving their interpretation in this unstructured manner the researcher is taking a qualitative approach to the study. However, as Field and Morse (1985) note, researchers need to take care that they maintain the focus of their study throughout in noting key aspects in an unbiased fashion. If, for example, a nurse researcher was observing the attitudes of nurses to their work-load she may note in general terms how temperatures were taken in the ward area but she would not attempt to apply measurements to these details in the same way as the nurse using a quantitative research method. Observational techniques give the researcher a great deal of scope in data collection. Rather than the limited approach of asking respondents how they would behave in a given situation that behaviour can be observed directly.

Specific observational techniques will be outlined in more detail below but before looking at that it will be useful to consider some factors that are encountered specifically by the researcher planning to use these techniques in their work.

Factors to consider before undertaking observation research

Observation techniques in research are time-consuming and are therefore a matter for careful consideration by researchers planning to utilise such techniques in research. Not only does the total time required have to be considered but the researcher needs to review how the time used for observations can be best used to facilitate the development of the study. Depending on the aim of the study it may be necessary to plan observational times around a 24-hour day in order to obtain a true picture of what is happening over that period when observing a particular situation. For example, a study of nursing work-load may be undertaken over 24 hours so that all factors affecting work-load over this time period may be considered in the research.

In addition to time other issues need to be carefully considered. In common with other research methods, the researcher must negotiate access to the intended site for the research. However, while organisations may readily give permission for a researcher to circulate a number of questionnaires among staff they may be less willing, for a variety of reasons, to give permission for a researcher to observe what is happening in particular environments. There may be anxieties about confidentiality in relation to situations observed. For example, there may be a risk of the researcher being placed in a difficult position if managers expect them to report on their findings in detail. Even if this is not a problem from a management perspective the staff being observed may themselves feel that the researcher has been put there to 'spy on them'. Obviously, all these issues must be considered very carefully before seeking permission to undertake the study and all staff must feel confident that their participation in any research study is on the understanding that confidences will not be breached.

Once the question of access has been addressed the researcher must consider other issues. They need to be sensitive to the impact of body language and recognise that the way in which they present themselves in their research capacity may affect the way in which information is shared. An aggressive approach (not one utilised by many researchers, it must be stressed) is hardly likely to generate confidence and a willingness to share among participants of observational studies. Included in the issue of presentation is the question of what to wear when observing. Again, this is dependent on the research design and the degree of participation involved in the study. At the outset the nurse researcher may feel it appropriate to wear a nurse's uniform. The problem with this is that it may create a situation when the nurse, in a ward area as an observer, may be expected to actually participate in care given. This may distort plans for a research project in which pure observational techniques are to be deployed. The option of what clothing to wear should be considered in relation to the specific study, but the researcher should aim as far as possible to be unobtrusive. Consequently, if carrying out an observational study in a ward area she may wear a white coat over her clothing to indicate that she is there in an official capacity. The nurse doing a community based study of the role of District Nurses and Health Visitors may, for example, be advised to wear smart everyday clothing.

Another issue that should be addressed is the possibility that when doing observational studies the researcher may experience role conflict. A nurse researcher undertaking a purely observational study in a very busy ward environment may feel guilty when trying to determine if she could do anything positive to help the nurses in their work. However, if she were to participate in the nursing activities this would have an effect on the situation being observed and introduce bias into the study. If the study was based on nursing work-load, for example, participation of the observer would have a direct impact on the work-load of other nurses in that area. Consequently, because nurses are so used to 'doing' nursing, a purely observational study can be a difficult approach for them to adopt. This should be considered in the initial planning and, if the nurse feels that she needs to participate in some way, she should plan for this in her research design.

Ethical issues should also be considered in observational approaches to research. For example, there is a remote chance that the researcher may observe situations which represent poor practices and so cause concern to the researcher. To interfere would, of course, affect the research study as a whole but nurses undertaking such projects must consider their own professional integrity when setting out as a researcher and determine at an individual level what action to take if faced with any difficult situations. Ultimately the safety of patients and staff must be of paramount importance.

The points above relate to the reactions of the observer to the research situation but it should also be noted that the people being observed may have their own reactions to the study. The classic problem associated with research of this kind is known as the Hawthorn effect, after a study undertaken in the USA in which this phenomenon was first observed. It was noted, in an experimental study, that awareness on the part of the subjects being studied had an effect on the dependent variable. This was related to the fact that participants saw themselves as being 'special' and so modified their behaviour in the course of the study. The importance of this to the researcher undertaking observational studies is that they must be aware of the possible impact that their presence may have on the research subjects and must, in their planning, consider ways in which any possible change of behaviour is avoided as far as possible.

In preparing for an observational study the researcher will spend a period of time becoming accustomed to the environment in which they plan to carry out the observations. The purpose of this is twofold. In the first instance it will allow those people in situations that are to be observed to become familiar with the fact that there is an extra person in their environment who appears to be taking note of what goes on. Allowing the research subjects time to become accustomed to the presence of a researcher will help to avoid any changes of behaviour that may occur as a result of being observed. It is generally accepted that after a period of familiarisation people forget that they are being observed in any way.

Secondly, the researcher will be able to develop their observational skills in readiness for the main study and perhaps give opportunity to test the research tool, if that has not been done already. It is because of these complex issues that a newcomer to nursing research would require considerable support when entering into a study requiring observational techniques. When looking at research projects that have utilised such approaches it is useful to read carefully how individual researchers have overcome the problems they faced.

Approaches to observational studies

As noted above, there are several possible variations to undertaking observational studies. These range from complete observer to acting as a participant observer. In all situations it is assumed that the researcher has sought and been given permission to undertake the research. There are reports of people undertaking research as a complete participant without advising anyone of the study in hand. Results published from such studies may lead to major protests because of the ethical implications of doing this. A nurse researcher might, for example, get a job as a nursing assistant for the purpose of studying that group in depth. It would be quite natural for the group of nursing assistants to react unfavourably if they found a researcher in their midst. Consequently, because of the ethical implications such approaches are positively discouraged in nursing research.

The ways in which a nurse could carry out observational research are outlined briefly here. The first of these is when a nurse acts as a *complete observer*. This technique is time-consuming and therefore should not be approached lightly. The researcher in this situation will have planned a very careful observational strategy and will take steps to ensure that they are able to observe relevant situations. For example, a researcher in a ward area may be there to observe the way that nursing staff practise aseptic techniques when applying abdominal dressings. As there are so many other activities in a ward at a given moment of time she must consider how best to observe these specific actions and how to exclude other, unrelated, activities from the observation. This can be done quite simply by devising some form of check-list on which the researcher will mark off any observations made in relation to aseptic techniques. Devising check-lists can be difficult so, as with other types of research, it is useful to seek the support of a supervisor in developing this. Also it is advisable to do a pre-test or pilot study to determine if the research tool is appropriate for the proposed study.

An alternative way in which a researcher could approach a study is to act as a *participant* in the area that they are observing. Researchers planning to perform observational studies are trying to acquire insight into the situation that they are observing and consequently may choose to assimilate with the study group for the purpose of the study. The method of data collection involving participant observation techniques was developed by anthropologists who were analysing behaviour in different cultures, hence some of the terms, such as ethnography and the use of field notes, that appear in research texts can be seen to originate from this type of work. If the researcher is working full-time on a project they may choose to act as a participant for the duration of the data collection part of the study. They could then be classed as an *observer working as a participant*. An alternative title, *participant as observer*, may be given if a member of staff chooses the observational method to research some aspect of practice in their own area of work.

Although the problems facing both observers and participant observers are similar there are potentially more ethical dilemmas involved in keeping records of activities of those staff that a researcher is working with. The problems facing the researcher undertaking this type of study relate both to the way in which they keep staff with whom they are working informed of their research activities and how they overcome the problem of keeping notes of their observations; many will admit to rushing off to the cloakroom to bring their field notes up to date. In addition, it is crucial that issues related to anonymity and confidentiality are clarified at the outset. The planning stage of the research study is crucial in identifying potential problems that may arise in the observation exercises and making strategy plans as to how to deal with these should they arise.

As with all studies the use of observational techniques in research will depend on the overall aims of the research project.

Summary

This chapter has explored some of the research methods available to nurses wishing to undertake studies of their own. It is not a definitive guide but rather a general outline of some of the methods frequently used by nurse researchers. The advantages and disadvantages of collecting information by using quantitative techniques have been discussed. Although it is acknowledged that there is an increasing interest in the subject of qualitative research, space allows only a limited exploration of this topic.

Case studies and action research have been briefly explored. Finally, the use of interviews, questionnaires and observational techniques in data collection have been outlined. In recognition of the limited space available to explore all of these issues readers wishing to undertake research studies are recommended to the further reading section below.

Further reading

Chenitz, W.C. and Swanson, J.M. (1986) *From Practice to Grounded Theory: Qualitative research in nursing*, Addison-Wesley Publishing, California.

Cohen, L. and Mannion, L. (1980) *Research Methods in Education*, Croom Helm, London.

Cormack, D.F.S. (1984) *The Research Process in Nursing*, Blackwell Scientific, Oxford.

Field, P.A. and Morse, J.M. (1985) *Nursing Reseach: The application of qualitative approaches*, Croom Helm, London.

Lathlean, J. and Farnish, S. (1984) *The Ward Sister Training Project*, NERU Report No. 3, University of London, London.

Leininger, M.M. (ed.) (1985) *Qualitative Research Methods in Nursing*, Grune & Stratton, Orlando.

Melia, K.M. (1982) ' "Tell it as it is": Qualitative methodology and nursing research: understanding the student nurses' world', *Journal of Advanced Nursing*, 7, 327–35.

Melia, K.M. (1987) *Learning and Working. The Occupational Socialisation of Nurses*, Tavistock Publications, London.

Moser, C.A. and Kalton, G. (1971) *Survey Methods in Social Investigation*, Heinemann Educational, London.

Oppenheim, A.N. (1966) *Questionnaire Design and Attitude Measurement*, Heinemann Educational, London.

Polt, D. and Hunglar, B. (1983) *Nursing Research. Principles and Method*, J.B. Lippincott, Philadelphia.

Treece, E.W. and Treece, J.W. (1986) *Elements of Research in Nursing*, 4th edn, C.V. Mosby, St. Louis.

8   Analysing research data

A short chapter on statistics has been included in this book simply as an introduction to the subject, in the hope that it may begin to demystify what may be seen as a very complex subject. Although there are a large number of people in society who have no difficulty in manipulating facts and figures, for many newcomers to research one of the most daunting challenges is that of understanding the use of statistics. The language can serve to confuse if the reader is not familiar with the terminology and consequently there can be a tendency to be suspicious of information presented in statistical form. As one of the reasons for using statistics is to present information in a manner that is easy to read and understand, any negative reaction to the subject should be overcome as quickly as possible. Some insight into statistics should serve to demystify the subject and make it seem less complex.

The purpose of statistics is to analyse measurements that have been made. If a nurse was doing a research study she would have decided what she wanted to measure when she defined her research problem. In designing the research tools she would be planning how she was going to measure the results. For example, she may design a questionnaire with a limited number of possible responses to each question asked, ranging from strong agreement to strong disagreement. She would anticipate collating these responses by counting the number to each option available; thus, she would be analysing the data. The purpose of statistics is to help the researcher to analyse data and to communicate the results in a form that represents shared understanding between the researcher and the reader. Statistics can be seen as a type of shorthand, giving a much quicker interpretation to facts and figures collated in a research study than by writing every detail in longhand.

As noted in the previous chapter, one way of collecting information in a quantitative study is by means of a questionnaire; this technique is commonly used to collect data for the purpose of description. By indicating the number and type of responses to a questionnaire when undertaking a survey the researcher can present results by using *descriptive statistics*. Descriptive statistics are a means by which the researcher can describe results in terms of their most important features.

A second approach is called *inferential statistics*. As the title implies, the statistics available may be used to 'infer' things about a population from the sample that has been studied. Unlike descriptive statistics, in which the information to be analysed is readily available and pertaining to a clearly defined situation, inferential statistics are used when there is a wish to generalise research findings from a sample of a given population to the whole of that population. The term used to describe this is statistical inference. This approach is normally utilised when undertaking an *experimental* or *correlational* study in which an attempt is made to predict some outcomes on the basis of the results from an experimental research study.

There are other ways in which results can be analysed and many factors that will impinge upon the methods used for statistical analysis. For further study of this subject the reader is referred to Hicks (1990) and other specialist texts noted in the reference section at the end of the chapter. The remainder of this chapter will focus on terms that may be commonly used in descriptive statistics and ways in which research data can be presented.

Descriptive statistics

When using statistics the researcher is trying to make sense of information that is available and to present it in some form that will be meaningful to others. There are many ways in which this can be done in everyday working life. For example, a nurse in the community may collect statistics relating to the number of elderly people in a small village community over a period of ten years. In collating these results she may note that the number of elderly people in that community had been steadily rising during that time span.

Similarly, a nurse on a ward may note the number of patients treated in that area in the course of the last month. She may compare that with the number of patients during the previous month and note that there is a radical difference. In following up this information the nurse may then obtain all the facts about the previous year's admissions to the area and decide to do more in-depth study into the fluctuations noted so that she can demonstrate changing trends to her managers. The hypothetical situations noted above provide a useful base from which to explore the subject of descriptive statistics further. Before looking at this it will be useful to explore ways in which information collected in this way can be presented.

Presenting research data

Tables

One of the most common means of presenting numerical information is to use tables which can summarise variables. Tables should be clearly labelled so

Table 8.1   Number of people over 75 years living in Groom

	Total	Men	Women
1980	28	15	14
1981	32	14	18
1982	33	14	19
1983	35	13	22
1984	32	13	19
1985	40	15	25
1986	49	17	22
1987	48	19	21
1988	55	25	30
1989	63	29	34
Total	415	174	224

Table 8.2   Diagnostic categories of admissions to Ward X during a 12-month period (n = 962)

	Bronchitis	Heart conditions	Neurological conditions	Other	Total
January	30	15	15	20	80
February	36	26	10	13	85
March	36	10	8	41	95
April	28	30	12	18	88
May	20	20	15	25	80
June	20	15	16	22	73
July	20	20	18	8	66
August	10	18	20	20	68
September	10	15	15	30	70
October	12	20	20	18	70
November	28	15	14	32	89
December	30	22	26	20	98
Totals	280(29%)	226(23%)	189(19%)	267(27%)	962(100%)

that the reader knows the purpose without having to scour the text for clarification. In addition they should be as simple as possible, as rows and rows of figures can be difficult for the reader to interpret. It is suggested in some statistical texts that it is better to have two simple tables than a single, complex one.

The community nurse mentioned above was collecting information about elderly people living in the community which has been called Groom. If Table 8.1 is reviewed it can be seen that it indicates how the total number of people over the age of 75 years has risen in that village community over the past ten years. The table also distinguishes the number of men and women represented in that group. Table 8.2 shows how the information the nurse in the hospital obtained has, in fact, given an indication of seasonal trends in the types of admissions in that medical ward area. There are far more admissions with bronchitis in the winter months. Another point useful to note at this stage is that a symbol commonly used to identify the total number of individuals or objects studied is 'n'. Hence, in Table 8.2 the symbols 'n = 962' indicate to the reader that the total sample for this study is 962 people. Abbreviations such as this allow tables to carry a lot of relevant information in a very limited space. The use of percentages in this table gives additional meaning to the results. The fact that 280 patients admitted with bronchitis represents 29% of the 962 patients admitted to the ward may be quite an important point for managers of health care planning to meet the needs of different groups of patients. The advantage to the researcher and subsequently the reader of presenting data in a numerical form is that it offers a type of shorthand, a very simple means of summarising a series of recordings or observations. The information in Tables 8.1 and 8.2 can be quickly reviewed and trends identified. If the nurses concerned had tried to write out in longhand what they had found in their studies the result would be a very lengthy document indeed.

The researcher presenting results from a study must have in mind the potential preferences of the reader when writing their report. There are some people who are able to interpret numerical information very quickly, while others need the implications to be spelt out clearly. In the majority of research reports note has been taken of this. Although there may be a scattering of tables of numerical values the interpretation of these results is spelt out in clear terms alongside. Tables are frequently used simply to support the points made in the written report.

There are several other ways in which the researcher can present data to make it easier for the reader to review by summarising key points. Of these the most commonly used are *graphs*, *histograms*, *bar charts* and *pie charts*.

Graphs

The use of graphs is familiar to all nurses: many aspects of nursing care are monitored using this approach. We record temperatures, pulses and respiratory rates using graphs. We may also use this format to record aspects such as weight, fluid intake or hours of sleep. We also use this information for comparison. For example, we may compare an increase in pulse rate with the temperature recording to identify if there are any identifiable trends. A rise in pulse rate noted may be associated with an increase in respiration or temperature. If this is not the case the nurse may consider other possible reasons for the increase in pulse rate. This normal, everyday practice for the

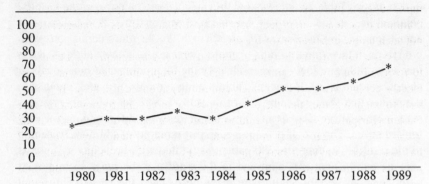

Figure 8.1   Graph showing number of elderly people in Groom

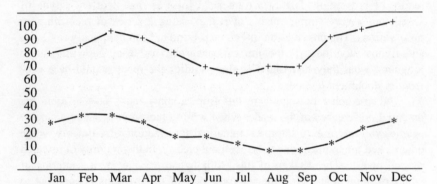

Figure 8.2   Graph showing number of patients admitted to medical ward as percentage of total admissions

* = Number of patients admitted with bronchitis
+ = Total number of patients admitted

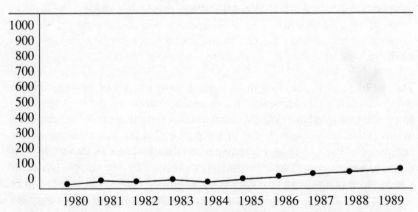

Figure 8.3   Poor graph design: showing the number of elderly people in Groom

nurse suggests that looking at graphs and analysing the observations noted is a common experience, an aspect that makes similar analysis in research terms not such a new experience for nurses.

To see how information can be translated into graph form it will be useful to review Figure 8.1. It can be seen that this graph indicates the number of elderly people living in the village community referred to above. It is very easy to see at a glance that there has been a rise in the elderly population over the ten year period studied; this information is contained in Table 8.2 but the graph offers stronger visual impact. Some of the information from Table 8.2 has also been converted into graph form. Figure 8.2 shows the number of patients admitted to the ward with bronchitis as a percentage of the total admissions. Again, it can be seen that although there are two groups identified in the graph the visual impact is more dramatic than the numerical data presented in Table 8.2 and offers a quick means of comparison between the groups represented.

In both Figures 8.1 and 8.2 it can be noted that in the graphs the horizontal axis has been used to record the time interval while the vertical axis has been used to note the frequency or number of observations made. It is accepted practice to present data in this way so that the frequency measure is along the vertical axis. It can also be seen that the range of figures used in the vertical axis is a realistic representation of the number of observations made. In Figure 8.1 the nurse did not take the number of years recorded beyond the time of her study or attempt to put large numbers over and above the sample studied in the horizontal axis. Had she done so the result might look something like Figure 8.3, a chart that does not support the information that is available to her, for the numbers are too small to be identified clearly in the numerical range given. This is a poor graph design, which may seem to be an obvious point and hardly worth noting in a book of this nature. However, it has been included purposefully to introduce a word of caution into the text. Inexperienced researchers may not use graphs well when sharing their knowledge. It is important when reading research reports that the information supplied in both axes of a graph is examined critically. It is very easy to show a line graph with very dramatic swings even when referring to very small samples.

Histograms and bar graphs

Histograms offer an alternative means of presenting information for instant visual impact. Information is presented in a series of vertical columns adjacent to one another. This allows the reader to note differences in information recorded. Figure 8.4 shows how this approach can be used to indicate the number of patients admitted to general hospital during a twelve month period.

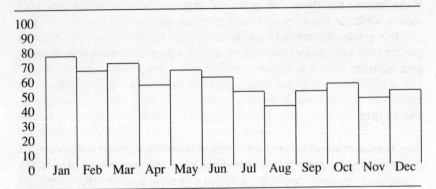

Figure 8.4   Histogram to show number of patients admitted to a general hospital during a 12-month period

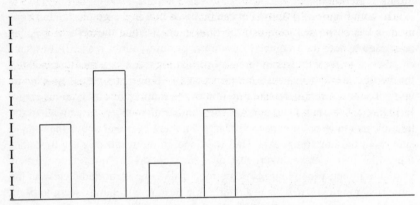

Figure 8.5   Example of a bar chart

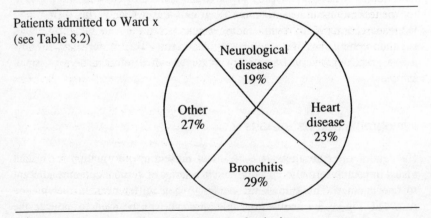

Figure 8.6   Example of a pie chart

It can be seen that there were more admissions in January than in any other month, while the lowest number occurs in August.

Bar graphs (Figure 8.5) are similar to histograms except that the data presented in the vertical bars are presented separately with spaces between each measure.

Pie charts

This is another popular way of presenting information for visual impact. As the name implies, presentation of information in this way can be likened to a pie: a circle is presented with slices to represent parts of the whole. An example of this format is noted in Figure 8.6, where the percentage of patient groups in Ward X (Table 8.2) is indicated. Although pie charts are a useful means of summarising information for visual impact it should be noted that it is not always easy to reflect data accurately in this approach, so it is perhaps used a little more cautiously by researchers than other methods of presentation.

There are other ways in which information may be visually presented following research projects, but those outlined above reflect those most commonly used. A good understanding of these basic principles will enhance the ability of those reading research reports to comprehend more complex patterns of presentation.

Measurements used in descriptive statistics

It has been noted earlier in this book that research studies utilising quantitative techniques are using some form of measurement. This means that the researcher needs to review measurement techniques available to analyse the data once it has been collected. The complexity of the analysis will vary depending on the complexity of the study, and the accuracy of the analysis will depend on the quality of the research tool and the data collection.

At a fairly simple level the use of percentages is a useful way of analysing data. For example, if a class of 50 student nurses in one school of nursing took an exam and of these 42 were successful the pass rate could be described as 84 per cent. Use of percentages also offers a simple way of comparing two groups of unequal size. If a second school of nursing in which of a group of 67 student nurses 51 students had passed the exam, the pass rate will be 76 per cent. The first group of students can therefore be seen to have a better pass rate than the latter.

Table 8.3   Number of patients admitted to
Ward Z during a 12-month period

Month	Patients (n)
January	26
February	35
March	15
April	33
May	18
June	22
July	10
August	11
September	12
October	16
November	14
December	28
Mean ($\bar{x}$) = 20 Total	240

Measures of central tendency

Several measures are commonly used in descriptive statistics, the use of which helps to interpret the meaning behind a set of results and offers an alternative way to tables, graphs and bar charts of presenting results. Measures of central tendency represent the results in terms of the most common features. Three terms are commonly used in these measures: mean, median and mode.

Mean

The *mean* is another word for the average. It is represented by the symbol $\bar{x}$. The sum of the observations is noted and divided by the total number of observations. To calculate the mean monthly admission rate using the data available in Table 8.3, the total number of patients admitted to Ward Z in a twelve month period would be calculated and divided by 12. Thus, the mean number of patients admitted to the ward is 20.

Of the three terms or measures of central tendency the mean is the most commonly used statistic, for it is more reliable and accurate than the others. This is because the mean depends on the value of every score and alteration in one score will have an impact on the mean. The disadvantage of using the mean, however, also lies in this factor since a radical change in just one score may have a dramatic effect on the mean. The mean does not give any information about the spread or distribution of scores. For example, if the number of patients admitted to Ward Z (Table 8.3) in June was reduced to 4 and the number of admissions in February was increased to 53 the mean score would remain at 26. However, the distribution of scores has changed in those months.

Median

The *median* represents a score that is mid-point in a set of results. If the total number of observations is arranged from the smallest to the largest the median represents what may be seen as the mid-point, in that half the scores are larger than and half are less than the median. For example, if the figures noted in a set of observations were

11,   20,   23,   27,   30,   33,   35   the median = 27.

If the number of observations noted is equal to an even number then the median is said to represent the mid-point between the two middle scores. In our example of patients in Table 8.3 there are twelve observations noted.

26   35   15   33   18   22   10   11   12   16   14   28

The two middle scores are 16 and 18; thus, the median would be 17.

One of the problems in using the median is that a given set of figures could be altered radically and yet the median remains the same. For example, in the numbers of patients noted above the highest number is 35. Were this changed to 350 the median would still remain the same. It can be seen, therefore, that the disadvantage of using the median is that it gives no information about the range of scores. It is unreliable and unstable as it could either be altered drastically by a single figure or not at all.

Mode

The *mode* is the expression used to describe the observation that occurs most frequently in the sample of data. In Table 8.3, when referring to the number of patients admitted, the mode can be seen to be 18. This is the number that occurs most frequently throughout the population noted and is the most common score. As with the median, the mode is seen to be an unreliable and unstable measure, for altering one figure drastically can have a major impact or no effect at all. In other words, it gives no information on how data is distributed. If the number of admissions noted in Table 8.3 was increased to 60 in January, February and March the mode would still be 18. If the number of admissions in May was increased to 35 the mode would change to 35.

The differences between the three measures should be noted, for incorrect use obviously undermines their potential value.

Measures of dispersion

The measures of central tendency have a limitation in that the mean, median and mode do not give a clear picture of how the data is spread. There is no indication as to whether the individual scores in a sample are close to the mean or are widely dispersed. This has practical implications in nursing situations. For example, a nurse manager may have been given the mean number of patients admitted to a ward area. Although a useful statistic, this alone may not help her in the deployment of staff for the number of admissions each week could change markedly and thus has implications for manpower planning. What this manager needs to know is the range of admissions to the unit. The statistics used to indicate this are known as measures of dispersion, for they are used to describe the distribution of data. Range, deviation and variance will be discussed below to illustrate the use of these measures.

Range

The *range* is a term used to describe the difference between the lowest and the highest value in a given set of figures. This is a useful measure, for it indicates the degree of difference between the two. To calculate the range the smallest score is subtracted from the highest. Thus, if the highest number of admissions to the ward in one week was 25 and the lowest was 2 the range would be calculated thus:

$$25 - 2 = 23.$$

The range is said to be 23. To illustrate this further let us look at the two sets of results produced by student nurses in their exams (Table 8.4). The range of

Table 8.4 Examination results: nursing students

	Group A	Group B
	44	10
	51	13
	52	20
	52	79
	50	90
	51	88
Total	300	300
Mean ($\bar{x}$) =	50	50

NB Pass mark = 45.

grades awarded in group A indicates that one student has failed to achieve the pass grade while in group B three out of six students have failed the exam. The range for group A results is 52–44=8. Group B range is 90–10=80.

A small range indicates a more homogenous set of data than a large range. This may be important. For example, an examiner comparing the range of the two sets of results would note the difference in scores between the two schools. The numbers of 6 and 80 as noted above do not mean very much on their own. There is a need to identify how the scores are distributed. To do this *deviation or variance* measures are used.

Deviation and variance

To calculate how far each set of scores deviates from the mean the mean is subtracted from each score, thus indicating the position of each score relative to the mean. If this is done with the results from students in groups A and B, the degree of deviation from the mean in both groups will be noted. Group A is obviously much closer to the mean (Table 8.5). Although the information in Table 8.5 gives a useful indicator of the deviation from the mean by the calculation of every score, it can result in presentation of data that appears complex and cumbersome. Consequently, it might be useful to group data to indicate the degree of variance for the group. This can be done by squaring each deviation score and totalling the products to achieve the *variance*.

Thus, if the results from the students in group A are computed,

$$(-6^2) + (1^2) + (2^2) + (2^2) + (0^2) + (1^2)$$
$$= 36 + 1 + 4 + 4 + 0 + 1$$
$$= \underline{46}$$

The variance figure represents the total variance of a set of scores, which indicates how dispersed or varied the scores are. The smaller the variance the more similar the scores. The greater the variance score the more disparate the results. To illustrate this point it may be useful for the reader to calculate the variance score for the students in group B and to compare the results with that noted above for group A students.

Table 8.5 Deviation from the mean ($x = 50$)

Group A	Group B
44–50 = –6	10–50 = –40
51–50 = +1	13–50 = –37
52–50 = +2	20–50 = –30
52–50 = +2	79–50 = +29
50–50 = 0	90–50 = +40
51–50 = +1	88–50 = +38

Standard deviation

This is the most important of the measures of dispersion for it represents the average or standard degree of deviation in a set of scores rather than the total degree of variation. If the amount of dispersion is large (as with the students in group B) so the standard deviation will have a greater numerical value. The formula used to describe the standard deviation can look frightening to the newcomer, but if broken down into component parts is not so difficult to understand.

$$SD = \sqrt{\frac{\Sigma (x - \bar{x})^2}{n}}$$

SD = standard deviation (sometimes written as s or o)
$\sqrt{}$ = square root of all the calculations under the symbol
(NB. The square root of a number x = the number which when multiplied by itself gives x, e.g. $\sqrt{}$ of 9 = 3 as 3 × 3 = 9)

$(\ )^2$ = squared number multiplied by itself (this is the variance score described above)
x = individual score
$\bar{x}$ = mean score
Σ = total sum
n = total number of scores in the sample group
(the symbol $n-1$ is used in inferential statistics when inferring information about the population from which the sample was taken. n is used when the SD from the sample only is used)

Normal distribution

For statistical purposes it is useful to know how the data is distributed graphically. One frequently occurring distribution is called normal distribution. Texts on statistics commonly use the example of height in the population to illustrate the point that when collecting data a pattern emerges that can be described as a 'normal' distribution.

If a large random sample of women living in the UK was taken, their weight measured and the results plotted on a graph, it is likely that the pattern that emerges on the page will be a bell shape. If the distribution was normal the mean, median and mode would be the same. This bell-shaped pattern is described as a normal distribution curve. It is useful in statistical terms, for it allows some degree of prediction to be made on the data gathered. In addition, some of the tests undertaken in inferential statistics rely on an assumption of

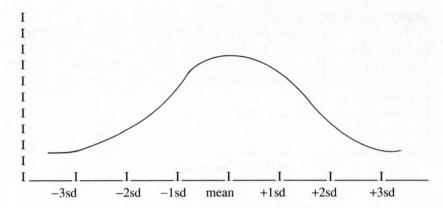

Figure 8.7   Normal distribution curve

normal distribution of data. The diagram in Figure 8.7 shows the normal distribution curve.

It can be noted that the standard deviation is marked on the diagram (Figure 8.7) and that a fixed percentage of scores in a set of normally distributed data fall within each standard deviation. In a normally distributed set of data 34 per cent of observations lie within one standard deviation on either side of the mean, therefore 68 per cent will always fall in this range. It is on this basis that the curve is useful in predicting what percentage of a population will fall into a given range.

It should be noted that not all data are normally distributed and other terms may be given to describe the pattern that emerges when results are plotted on a graph. A *skewed* distribution can be described as a positive or negative pattern. Figure 8.8 shows a positive skew. Such a pattern may occur if an examination paper at the end of the first year of a nursing course was too difficult for the student group. Figure 8.9 shows a negative skew. This may be demonstrated if the end-of-year examination was too easy for the student nurses. A *bimodal* distribution can also occur. Figure 8.10 indicates the type of pattern that might emerge if the same examination was set for student nurses in their first and third years of training. It would be expected that the third-year group would achieve higher grades. A J-shaped curve (Figure 8.11) can occur if, for example, the pulse rate was recorded a few minutes after students had run around the building as part of an applied physiology session. It would be expected that, if the students were fit, the pulse rate would be high when they stopped running but fall to normal in a very short time after the exercise. However, it is likely that a few less fit individuals will retain a higher pulse for a longer period.

It is useful to appreciate these terms, for they may be used in research texts when describing the range of results obtained in a study.

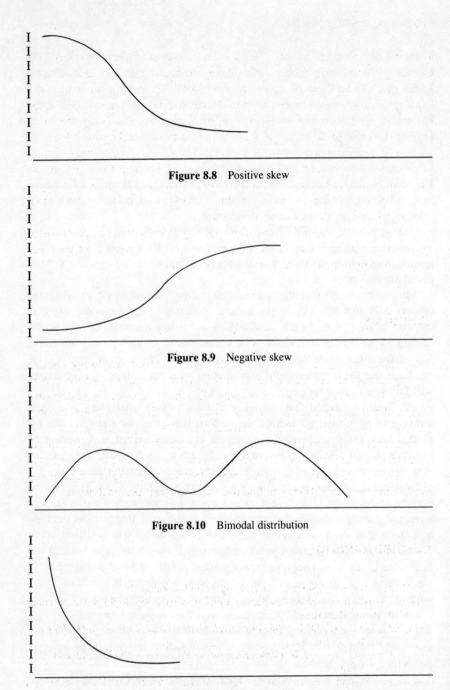

Figure 8.8   Positive skew

Figure 8.9   Negative skew

Figure 8.10   Bimodal distribution

Figure 8.11   J-shaped curve

Computers and research

It should be noted briefly that computers are a useful resource to researchers planning to undertake statistical tests. Many computer firms produce software packs that can be used to analyse research data. These have proved to be a great time-saver for anyone wishing to do statistical testing in research. If the researcher wishes to take advantage of such packages this issue should be considered early in the planning stage of the study so that the research design matches the facilities available for analysis. The rate of development of computer technology is such that it is advisable to ask for help from experts, for they will be able to advise on most recent developments. The nurse wishing to use computers to help to analyse research findings could seek advice from staff in regional or district computer centres.

In addition to the use of statistical packages computers can be of use to nurses interested in research, for there are an increasing number of packages available to help to facilitate learning about research.

Summary

This chapter has given an overview of descriptive statistics exploring some of the key issues that are relevant to both the reader of research and the person planning to undertake a small-scale study. Methods of presentation of data have been outlined and measures of central tendency and dispersion discussed. It is recognised that understanding of statistics causes much anxiety to nurses, so consequently the further reading section has been kept to a minimum. There are an increasing number of books on statistics available and if the reader wishes to take study of this further it is recommended that they explore the options available in their local library to find one that suits their personal needs.

Further reading

Day, C. (1985) *From Figures to Facts*, King's Fund, London.

Hicks, C. (1990) *Research and Statistics: A practical introduction for nurses*, Prentice Hall, Hemel Hempstead.

Reid, N.G. and Boore, J.R.P. (1987) *Research Methods and Statistics in Health Care*, Edward Arnold, London.

Treece, E.W. and Treece, J.W. (1986) *Elements of Research in Nursing*, 4th edn, C.V. Mosby, St Louis.

Woodward, M. and Francis, L.M.A. (1988) *Statistics for Health Management and Research*, Edward Arnold, London.

9   Sharing research knowledge

Nurses undertaking research studies frequently experience more anxiety over the issues addressed in this chapter than any other part of their research studies. Because of this, and because sharing knowledge is seen to be a crucial part of the research process, this chapter has been included in this book. The section on writing skills explores aspects of writing that may be demanded of nurses undertaking research studies. Skills of presentation have been included because it is now fairly common practice for nurses who have undertaken research studies to be asked to share their ideas, experiences or research results with their colleagues in a formal presentation.

Writing skills

The anxieties experienced at the thought of doing written work is not uncommon and newcomers to research often require more help with writing about their work than with any other part of the study. Although it must be acknowledged that some people have more of a natural flair for writing than others, one reason why people might underestimate their ability to write well may simply be due to lack of practice. For many nurses approaching research studies for the first time it may have been some years since they were required to produce a formal piece of written work. The purpose of writing is to convey ideas from one mind to another. If the nurse is to do this successfully and present written work in a way that is meaningful to the reader there are some guidelines that can help. These apply whether writing an essay, a research proposal, a research report or an article for publication.

Essay writing
It is common practice for students undertaking research studies to be asked to produce an essay for their first piece of assessed work. The purpose of this is twofold. In the first instance it allows the student to begin to practice the writing skills required for the course. Secondly, it allows the teacher to assess

the student's ability to write at the academic level required on the particular course of study, while also assessing the individual student's level of understanding of the given topic. Because of this approach in research courses some general guidelines for essay writing are outlined below.

Planning

The planning stage is crucial in the writing process and yet it is one that is often neglected. Quite commonly, in poor essays the writer has no obvious systematic plan and the overall structure of the piece of work is poor. If the writer changes from one subject to another in an erratic fashion, the reader may be unable to understand the ideas presented in the essay. The writer may be clear in their own mind as to what they want to say yet they are failing to do this in a way in which the reader can understand.

When planning an essay it is useful to follow some very simple guidelines:

1. Be sure that the topic of the essay is clearly understood. It is easy to become side-tracked when writing essays and if this happens the writer may fail to address the title of the essay. It is useful to highlight relevant points in the title or question by underlining them. As work is being prepared it is useful to keep asking whether key issues are being addressed.

2. Read any relevant literature pertaining to the subject. When reading take notes, or underline, any relevant factors that could be included in the essay. The amount and nature of the literature read at this stage will depend on the academic requirements of the course. If a nurse is undertaking a master's degree programme the expectation will be higher than if she was doing an essay as part of a short course of study into the research process.

3. Following this think about the topic in detail and consider all relevant aspects that may be discussed. At this stage make note of the order of priority that will be given to the points raised. In so doing, *write a plan*.

4. Review the plan and consider whether there are clearly defined sections and if the sequence of information is logical.

5. Write a *draft essay*. This is a very important stage when essay writing. The student who is able to produce a perfect piece of work at a first attempt is a very rare breed indeed. Although some of us may aspire to such ability it is far more common for good pieces of written work to have undergone several revisions before the writer feels that they have fully completed the work.

A useful tip at this stage is to write the essay on one side of the paper only. This will allow the order, or structure, of the essay to be changed if, on revision, it is felt that the work does not flow logically from topic to topic. The order can be simply changed by cutting out the relevant sections of the essay and transferring them to a more appropriate spot. (Glue or tape can be useful here.)

Another useful tip is to write on alternate lines, or at least leave plenty of space between the lines of writing. This will enable corrections to be made in such a way that work can be read when the amendments are done.

An increasing number of people now have access to word processors. These can be a valuable tool when writing and editing work and can, in the long term, save much energy when reviewing draft documents.

There are several advantages to writing a draft copy. The first is that the writer will be able to scrutinise their work critically to see if the plan has been followed and that the meaning is clear. Secondly, in writing a draft copy the writer has some information at hand to share with a supervisor or teacher who will be able to give advice on how to progress. If a teacher is not available there may be a colleague who is prepared to give peer support and comment constructively on a draft essay. Alternatively, it is useful to pace essay writing in such a way that once the draft copy has been completed, it can be put to one side for a few days. The writer can then return to the work and review it themselves. It is frequently the case that a break from written work helps the writer to approach it from a fresh perspective and see it more from a 'reader's eye'. When reviewing a draft copy the following points should be considered:

(a) The introduction should be clearly related to the essay title and clarify any issues within that. Any ideas or concepts that will be used in the essay should be stated and some indication given as to the depth in which issues will be explored in the essay. This can be done in a brief overview of the content of the essay.

(b) The structure of the essay should then be analysed. It should be noted first whether the essay progresses logically and systematically. If this is so then each paragraph will be written around a theme or sub-theme. Sentences should be simple and related to one idea only. Arguments for and against points made should be clearly stated and appropriate evidence given to support points made. An academic essay should not be a collection of unsupported opinions; it should be a well-reasoned and balanced discussion in which issues are discussed in an objective and critical manner.

(c) The use of literature in the text should be appropriate and the writer should clearly note when they have used information from other sources. Failure to do this may be interpreted as plagiarism. Some key points relevant to referencing information in an essay are outlined below:

(i)   If a direct quote is used from another source indent the lines used and use quotation marks. In printed texts the line spacing, and or letter size, may be altered to ensure that the quotation stands out clearly from the main body of the text.

> This quote has been directly copied from a book on the art of nursing research and consequently has been presented in this format on this page.

(ii) If ideas from another source are used, but not the exact words of the original author, the information, or ideas, can be incorporated into the writing and credit to the source material given at end of the account.

Other methods that may be used for referencing such material are noted in more detail in Chapter 6. In summary, the writer may choose to make reference by indicating the name of the author and the date of publication at the end of the section, i.e. (Bloggs, 1989). This is known as the Harvard system. Alternatively, they may choose to use the numerical approach of indicating references in which names and dates are not necessarily included in the text but listed by number at the end of the paper. This is known as the Vancouver system.

(d)   The writing style is important when writing academic essays; they are generally written in the third person. One of the difficulties when writing in the first person is that it personalises work in such a way that it is not evident to the reader that the writer is presenting information objectively. If the writer were to say 'I think nursing research is . . . ' it does not indicate that others may also have identified similar trends. Statements such as 'It has been suggested that nursing research is . . . ' or 'there is evidence to suggest that nursing research is . . . ' can be used to overcome this and to present written work in a more objective fashion. The writer should take care to ensure that a consistent approach is used throughout the essay.

(e)   When writing essays the use of complicated jargon should be avoided. A good guide is never to use a complicated word, or number of words, when a simple one will make the point just as well. This word of caution is particularly important for prospective researchers, as one of the reasons given in Chapter 2 for failure to spread research findings is that the language used may be too complex for many practitioners to understand. Although there are occasions when it is difficult to avoid technical language the writing should always be presented in a way that is meaningful to the audience it is being prepared for.

(f)   The conclusion of an essay should be unambiguous and relate clearly to the content of the essay. The writer should refer back to the points made in the introduction, summarise what has been said about these in the discussion and base the final conclusion on the evidence that has been presented in the essay.

(g) A full reference list should accompany the essay. The purpose of this, as noted above, is to give credit to any other work incorporated into the essay. In addition the reference list gives a source of information to the reader wishing to explore ideas highlighted in the work.

6. *Completing the essay:* only when a thorough editorial review, or critique, of the draft essay has been done is the student ready to write the final piece of work. All the points noted above should have been considered. The end result, the completed essay, should be a neat, logical and well-balanced piece of work.

Writing for research

If the nurse has mastered the skills required for writing a good academic essay she will easily be able to transfer that knowledge to writing for research. Specific areas that will be explored in this section are writing both a research proposal and a research report. Before we explore these, however, it is worth outlining briefly what is expected in a literature review, for this is crucial to any writing for research.

Literature review

A literature review may be undertaken for a variety of reasons, as identified in Chapter 6. For example, this may be used to support the rationale for undertaking or replicating a research study. In addition, it is common practice for nurses learning about research to be asked to undertake a literature search and to write a review of this as part of their course work. Searching for literature is covered in some detail in Chapter 6 and will not be examined here. The focus in this section will be on the written report, the literature review.

The first thing to clarify when writing a literature review as part of a course-work assignment is to determine the required length of the work and the expected completion date. If a 1000-word assignment has to be produced in a four-week period then the detail in the work will not be expected to compare with a literature search incorporated in a Ph.D. thesis. This may seem to be an obvious statement but all too often the students undertaking a literature search for the first time become involved with the subject and gather so much information that it is impossible to utilise this adequately in a written review. The skills of synthesising knowledge can be developed with practice.

It is not true that the more references available in a piece of work the better it is. Sometimes the reverse is true, for too much information may only serve to confuse. What is important is that relevant information is used well. Quality, not quantity, is a good guide when preparing a literature review.

The literature review should have an introduction, a discussion section and a conclusion. The introduction should inform the reader of the subject area, how the literature search was undertaken and what sources of information were utilised in this. For example, the *International Nursing Index* may have been used or an on-line (computer) search instigated. The volume of research material in some subject areas is enormous and the writer will need to clarify in the introduction exactly what constraints they have faced and what measures have been taken to overcome them. For example, the volume of research work undertaken into pressure area care is large; consequently, a review of literature in this area may be specific, focusing perhaps on one particular treatment.

The literature review should clearly relate to the area of research interest. Previously published research on the subject should be analysed and summarised. When reading a wide range of literature on a topic it is commonly found that specific views, or themes, can be identified. All views should be represented in an unbiased literature review. Both sides of an argument, or conflicting research results, should be presented, even if they conflict with the writer's own beliefs on a subject.

The conclusion to a literature review can be short but should, as in essay writing, summarise the key points. A full and accurate reference list should be available at the end of the literature review.

Research proposal

It was noted in Chapter 4 that it may be necessary to write out a research proposal prior to undertaking a study. The reason for this may be that the researcher is applying for financial support to fund the study or they may be seeking permission from an ethical committee to undertake the work. Nurses undertaking research courses may be asked to prepare a research proposal as part of the course requirements to demonstrate their understanding of the research process. Even if there is no formal demand on the researcher to write a proposal prior to the study it is a useful exercise, for it helps to focus onto the key issues in the research and facilitates the planning of the study in providing a structured outline of intent. Before preparing a research proposal it is important that the requirements of the 'audience' it is being written for are clarified, as the approach may differ slightly. Many organisations offering grants for research purposes have their own format for research proposals. The same is true of some ethical committees. It is in the researcher's own interest to follow the preferred style of the group to which they are presenting the research proposal.

Table 9.1 Comparison between a research proposal and a research report

Research proposal	Research report
Future tense	Past tense
Title	Title

Introduction
  Background to study
  Aims/hypothesis
	Introduction
	  Background to study
	  Aims/hypothesis

Literature review – outline	Literature review – full

Methodology
  Proposed
	Methodology
	  Actual

Details relevant to application
  Time
  Funding
  Staff involved
	Results
	  Analysis of data

Conclusion	Discussion
	  Conclusions
	  Limitations of study
	  Recommendations

	References Appendix (optional)

The presentation of the research proposal is another important point. Every effort should be made to avoid using complex jargon; it will not help the application if the committee approving the proposals have difficulty in understanding the subject. In general terms, the research proposal follows the stages of the research process and so there are similarities with a research report. The research proposal is, however, written in the *future tense* while the research report would be written in the *past tense*. The following guidelines outline the presentation of a research proposal. These are summarised in Table 9.1.

The *title* of the research proposal study should clearly reflect the subject of the study. It is tempting to spend time thinking of good literary titles for proposed research studies but these may have little value in future indexing of the work. For example the title 'Bad Experience' may catch the eye in a shelf of fictional books but it will not tell future nurse researchers that the contents reflect a study of communication in hospital settings.

The *introduction* to the research proposal should clearly state the background to the proposed study indicating why there is a need for this particular work to be done. This will set the proposed study into a suitable context for discussion. The implications of undertaking the study could also be identified at this stage.

The *aims, or hypothesis*, of the study should then be stated to clarify the specific purpose of the research. It may be necessary to define any terms that are being used in the context of the study at this stage.

The *literature review* is the next step. Although this may not be demanded as a separate section in all research proposals, a review of the literature serves to support the rationale for undertaking the research. It may be kept brief, simply outlining some of the key work related to the subject area and the relevance of this to the proposed study.

The next area to consider is the proposed *research method*. In this section the research design should be described. The population and study sample should be identified. Anticipated ethical dilemmas, issues related to confidentiality and access to research sites should be outlined. Any proposed measurement device, such as questionnaires, should be identified and a rationale given for this choice. The method of data collection should be described and the proposed method of analysing data noted. If the researcher has already prepared a research tool, for example a draft questionnaire, for the study it is helpful to include this in an appendix attached to the proposal.

The information above represents the basic requirements for a research proposal. The researcher seeking support in terms of funding and, perhaps, time to do the study, will need to include more detail in their proposal. A full account of anticipated expenditure and the time required to undertake the investigation should be noted. It may be necessary to give more detail about the staff to be involved in the research study, particularly if a research assistant is to be employed. Applicants may also be asked to submit a curriculum vitae with their research proposal, for this will give any selection committee an indicator as to whether the applicant has the appropriate background to undertake the study as proposed.

As with all other pieces of written work it may be appropriate to write a brief conclusion. This could be used to emphasise important points and to reinforce the perceived value in undertaking the study proposed.

Research report

The pattern adopted to write a research report reflects that used to write a research proposal (see Table 9.1). The report is written in the past tense and obviously contains more detail than a research proposal, as all aspects of the research process will be discussed.

In the section on research proposals three sections were identified: an introduction, in which the aims or hypothesis are clearly stated and the background to the study explained; a review of the literature; and a section on proposed methodology. When writing the research report the researcher would elaborate on all these sections. Confidentiality should be maintained throughout the research report.

The *results* of the study will be presented. The volume of data included in this section is left to the discretion of the researcher. Although it may be seen as ideal to exhibit all the data gathered during the course of a research study, this may cause the text to become too complex. To overcome this researchers frequently use tables and graphs, as these offer a shorthand way of presenting data. An alternative approach is to summarise findings and include the results in appendices at the end of the research report so that data is available for reference purposes.

If the researcher has stated an hypothesis they may state in the section giving the research results whether it has been accepted or rejected. Otherwise the presentation of results is simply a description of findings. The advantage to readers of research reports is that they can read this section objectively to determine what they feel to be the outcome of the research.

The final section in a research report is the *discussion*. At this point the researcher discusses the results obtained in the context of the aims of the research, the research setting and in relation to any other background information highlighted in the literature review. Aspects related to the research methodology can be highlighted, with specific emphasis placed on any particularly interesting results. Within the final discussion the researcher should acknowledge any limitations to the study that may have affected the final outcome.

Finally, the researcher will consider any recommendations they wish to make as a result of the study. This may, for example, be a recommendation specifically related to the subject of the research, or alternatively to research design in future studies. Many research studies leave the researcher with more questions than answers, and it is not uncommon for the closing lines of a research report to indicate a need for further study into an area of practice.

At the end of a research report will be a list of *references*. If the researcher has used material to create an *appendix* this would complete the report and be included after the reference section. The appendices are generally used to hold any information seen as relevant to the study as a whole but not so essential that they should be incorporated in the main text. For example, letters asking for permission to undertake a study are not necessarily included in the text of a report but are important to refer to when describing the methodology. Also, as noted above, it may be distracting to put all the research data into a report, yet this may need to be available for reference purposes.

The information outlined above provides a general guideline for writing research reports. Examination of many published research texts will reveal that, although the format noted above will be identifiable in some reports, others will have a different structure. Ultimately the researcher will plan the specific format of their report based on the structure of their overall research study.

Writing for publication

All nurses who undertake research studies need to consider how to share their findings with their colleagues. One obvious way to reach a wide audience is to prepare a research report for publication. The following information is given as a guideline for nurses who may wish to publish their research work.

The first thing to decide is to which journal to submit their paper, as this helps to clarify the audience for which the article is being written. If this is not done a paper may need to be rewritten to meet the needs of the target audience of a particular journal. All journals produce their own guidelines for contributors. In many journals these are included on the back page of each copy, while for others there may be a need to write to the editor for information. The journal guidelines advise on the length of the article, the writing style, the preferred referencing system and the presentation of tables and graphs. It is normal practice for journals to request at least two manuscripts which have been typed with double spacing. This is to facilitate editorial work.

It may be worth contacting the editor before writing an article to determine whether there would be sufficient interest to publish the paper. If the researcher has explored a specialist subject area, for example, it may not be seen as relevant to a journal with general readership. Alternatively, if the editor feels that a particular topic has received sufficient coverage in recent months they may not be interested in publishing another report on the topic at this moment. If this is known at the outset it can save much time and energy for both the writer and the reviewer.

When writing for publication the guidelines given in the previous section still apply and a similar format is followed. If writing a research report for publication, however, the researcher would need to consider the emphasis that is placed on each section of the report. It may be necessary for them to determine priorities in selecting material for inclusion in the article and the weighting given to each section may need to be adjusted to match the word limit of the finished article. The length of journal articles varies, but 2–3,000 words is a fairly average length for publication.

In any article submitted for publication particular note should be taken of anonymity. In offering research subjects confidentiality when undertaking studies the researcher should ensure that this is not breached by a slip of the pen in preparing an article. It is a useful exercise to read some research reports in journals to see how confidentiality is maintained in these. In so doing a pattern can be identified in which terms such as 'A Health Centre in the Midlands' or 'A group of nurses in a large teaching hospital' are used to give anonymity, while also setting into context the location of the study.

The researcher would be expected to write an abstract to accompany the article. This is a short summary of the project and should give a succinct overview in approximately 150 words. In this the purpose and results of the study should be made clear to the reader. The value of an abstract is that it allows the reader to determine whether the contents of a paper are relevant to them.

It is also a matter of courtesy for the writer to consider any support, help or co-operation that has been received during the course of the study. This may have been from research subjects, a supervisor or a source of funding given to the study. It is accepted practice to acknowledge such support given at the end of an article.

When articles are submitted for publication the writers are advised to keep a copy. This is essential in the first instance because papers can be lost in transit and, if that were to happen without another copy being retained, all the hard work involved in preparation would be wasted. A second good reason for keeping a copy is that when an article is published it is useful to review how much editorial work has been done on it. This will help the writer to gauge their own skills in writing for this medium and may therefore be a useful learning experience.

Writers are not advised to submit the same work to more than one magazine at a time, as this can lead to complications in the area of copyright if the work is accepted for publication. Once an article has been submitted for publication the writer should be prepared for a long wait before final confirmation of acceptance or rejection. Most journals operate a system of review in which articles are sent out to a professional panel who determine suitability for publication. This system does have positive benefits but it is quite a time-consuming process. If the journal accepts an article they may do so provisionally, dependent on some modification, or they may accept it as it is. Once it is accepted the writer is asked to sign a contract which clarifies issues related to publication and copyright of the material when published.

Pubishing material is not an easy process, for there is much demand on a limited amount of space. Consequently, researchers need to consider other ways in which information can be shared. As this includes presenting information verbally the next section concentrates on presentation skills.

Presentation skills

This section has been included in a book on research because of the responsibility held by the researcher to ensure that research findings are shared with as wide an audience as possible. Before exploring this topic it is worth stressing that anyone interested in undertaking research of their own must anticipate that there will come a time when they will be expected to share their findings in a seminar or lecture format. The skills of verbal presentation can be developed with practice. It is hoped that the information included in this section will help newcomers to research to develop the skills required to share their knowledge with others in a meaningful way.

It is not unusual for nurses asked to speak publicly for the first time to experience extreme anxiety. However. following the first experience most will admit that they have gained a lot of confidence. A little anxiety before public speaking is seen by some to be important, for this can be constructive and helps to motivate the speaker towards a more polished performance. If the speaker does not feel some anxiety they may demonstrate an over-confident approach that can lead to a poor presentation. There is no doubt that public speaking is a nerve-racking experience but anxieties related to this can be markedly reduced if the speaker is well prepared, and so the following sections give guidelines on the skills required to give a good presentation.

Preparing a lecture

The principles of presenting information apply regardless of the subject matter, be that a research report or a lecture on a more general subject area. For convenience the term 'lecture' is used in this section to illustrate the points made in relation to presenting information to a group. Where appropriate, information specific to the presentation of research papers will be given.

Organisational factors

1.   The first step in preparation is to clarify the topic of the lecture. It is important to ensure that the speaker and the organiser have the same expectation of the content of the talk. If a timetable for the day is available this can be consulted to ensure that there is no overlap with subject area and the presentation of any other speaker. If there are areas of similarity it is important that these are discussed at an early stage in preparation so that any repetition of subject material is avoided.

2.   Clarify how much time is allocated for the presentation. Lecture time allocated can vary. An hour is a fairly common time period for many situations to which researchers are invited to share their findings with small groups. However, if presenting a research paper at a conference the time allocated may be only 15 minutes and it is obviously crucial that this is known beforehand. In conferences that are tightly scheduled for time it is normal for the chairman to stop the speaker when the allocated time is used. If the speaker was not fully prepared for this they might not have got beyond the introduction. It is even harder for a speaker to be prepared for 15 minutes and find that the organisers expect the session to last an hour.

3. Make sure that the audience 'mix' is known. This allows the speaker to adjust the presentation to match the level of knowledge of the audience. It may be assumed, for example, that there is a different level of knowledge in a group of trained staff compared with a group of nurses who have just begun their course of training. If the level of presentation is inappropriate then the audience can become restless and this can be most distracting for the speaker.

4. Identify the venue of the lecture. This is probably best done nearer the time of the lecture but is included here as a relevant organisational factor. If possible, identifying the venue of the lecture may give the opportunity to explore the facilities available before speaking.

It is useful to check the acoustics in the room, if possible. If it is a large area it may be useful for the speaker to take a friend or colleague to sit on a back row to see if they can hear the presentation in a full rehearsal. There may be a need to practice voice projection, for example. Alternatively, if there is a microphone available it would be helpful to practice using this so that it is a familiar tool by the time the lecture commences.

If travelling some distance to give a lecture some of these points may have to be checked on the day. However, it is important to check travel arrangements and parking facilities if appropriate as a last-minute rush can cause added anxiety.

Preparing the lecture paper

Having clarified the organisational aspects the researcher can concentrate on preparing the paper for presentation. The principles of public speaking are the same as writing. When preparing a paper for a lecture the introduction should 'set the scene'; the main body of the talk should discuss key issues; the conclusion should summarise what has been said.

If giving an outline of a research project the nurse will need to determine priorities, for if allocated a short time it may not be sufficient to cover all aspects of a study. A source of reference for an audience can do much to reduce the frustrations that occur as a result of time limitation for a presentation. For example, it may be possible to refer the audience to the original research report which may be available in an unpublished format. Some libraries in schools of nursing keep copies of work for this purpose.

When preparing material for a lecture it is fairly common for the first draft to include too much detail; this is not a bad thing, for it serves to ensure that the knowledge base of the speaker is wide. This helps the individual level of confidence, particularly when questions are invited from an audience.

Following critical review of the draft content the lecture should be adjusted to match the time available. The key headings should be clearly identified and the method of presentation considered.

Method of presentation

Speakers are generally invited to talk on a topic that reflects an area of special interest to them. This makes both preparation and presentation easier, for interest tends to inspire enthusiasm. It is important, however, to beware of an overenthusiastic approach for this too can be detrimental to a presentation.

The key factor in considering how to present a lecture is to think of ways in which the interest of the audience can be retained. It is useful for anyone involved in presenting information to note the strengths and weaknesses of any lecture sessions that they have attended. This usually gives clues as to what may be considered good techniques to adopt. The points noted below are not exhaustive by any means, but contain some useful tips for the newcomer to public speaking:

1. It is not generally advisable to read the paper, word for word, to an audience. On occasion this approach works quite well, but frequently the result is a presentation which does little to capture the imagination of the audience. A compromise can be reached by identifying key headings from a written paper and using these to guide the presentation. If this is done the result is likely to be a more relaxed approach as long as the presenter does not try to memorise word for word what is written on the paper. Audio-visual aids can be used to help to remember detail and to explain more complex issues, such as research results. The use of these will be discussed in more detail later.

2. It is useful to rehearse a presentation beforehand; a tape recorder helps with this for it is possible to check back and critically review the content of the lecture. Of course, it is never quite the same rehearsing in the privacy of the home environment as in front of an audience, but a rehearsal can certainly help to exclude those words or awkward phrases that are likely to cause problems when speaking in public. In addition it might inspire the speaker to change the tone of voice if the presentation sounds monotonous on tape; the timing of a presentation can be adjusted as this type of rehearsal allows speakers to check on how long their presentation lasts.

3. Jargon should be avoided. When presenting information the same advice on the use of jargon as that given in the section on writing skills applies. Do not use complex words when a simple one will do. The use of jargon can serve to alienate the speaker from the audience. If presenting a research paper it is important to remember that what might be everyday language to a researcher will not necessarily be so to an audience.

4.   Body language is another important point to consider, for this tends to give the audience clues about the individual presenting the paper. Experts suggest that body language is more honest than verbal communication and gives a much stronger source of information than the spoken word. To illustrate this it might be useful to consider the reaction of an audience listening to a speaker talking about communication skills and yet failing to look at the audience while speaking. As one of the key aspects in good communication is maintaining eye contact the non-verbal cues received by the audience in this situation may not match the content of the lecture. This is a key factor that must be considered. The speaker should, of course, face the audience and should aim, as far as possible, to maintain eye contact with that group. This may not be easy for the newcomer to lecturing but it does become easier with practice.

Other traits should be considered. For example, do not point at people, do not stand with arms folded, do not turn your back on the audience. All these are distancing gestures. In addition, mannerisms that may be seen as irritating by your audience should be avoided. Twiddling with a curl of hair, for example, may be a mild mannerism but can be irritating to an audience if it distracts them from the content of the presentation.

5.   Ways of encouraging audience participation can be considered. Anecdotes can increase audience participation and change their role from a passive to an active one. They should, however, be used with caution for they can be distracting when presenting factual material. If the speaker has the confidence, and opportunity allows, questioning the audience can increase participation and serve to sustain interest. This approach is perhaps only of use to smaller audiences.

There are many tricks of the trade adopted by teachers to maintain the interest of their audience. Such skills are seen as essential in teaching for there is evidence to suggest that when listening to lectures concentration cannot be sustained for a long period. Consequently, it is useful to consider ways in which the key points of any lecture can be made clear to the audience. Although, with practice, public speakers can do much to enhance the liveliness of their verbal presentation and so retain interest, the use of audio-visual aids offers an excellent medium by which points can be clarified and audience concentration focused.

Audio-visual aids

In this modern world the scope and variety of audio-visual aids available is tremendous, ranging from the chalk board to computer technology. When presenting a lecture, however, speakers must feel confident with any equipment used and this does, to some extent, limit the range of audio-visual aids that can be utilised by the newcomer to public speaking. Consequently the following discussion will only focus on a few of the more popular visual aids used. It should be stressed at the outset that audio-visual aids are of benefit only if they are used well; if speakers have any doubt about their ability they may be better advised to limit their use until more practised. However relevant or interesting a talk, inappropriate use of visual aids can distract an audience in such a way as to spoil the reception of the information by the audience.

Chalk board

The chalk board has been a common sight in classrooms for many years and still remains a popular tool in teaching. Traditionally the term 'blackboard' is used but as modern technology takes over and we have available white boards, on which coloured ink pens are used, different names will be used to describe a similar visual aid. The advantages of using boards of any sort is that it allows the lecturer to note key points as they arise in the presentation, to indicate how issues are linked by illustration and to demonstrate more clearly factual material. Information noted on the board should be minimal with only key points noted. For example, a researcher may use this medium to highlight a few key results following a research study. It is not correct use to attempt to write out a potted version of lecture notes.

The first disadvantage of using a board is that it requires a moderate amount of confidence on the part of the lecturer. Thinking about what to write at the same time as concentrating on what is being said can be quite a complex process. If used inappropriately this tool can serve to alienate the speaker from the audience; first, because it is difficult to write without the speaker turning their back on the audience. Secondly, if they are not able to write clearly and concisely the effort made to use the board may be wasted as the audience may cease to concentrate on what is being said, trying instead to translate the symbols on the board.

In relation to this last point, chalk boards are generally only of use if speaking to fairly small groups, for all members of the audience should be able to read what has been written without any difficulty. If speakers find themselves with a large group and only this medium for illustration then they should make minimal use of the board and adjust the size of their writing to ensure that all of the audience can see what has been written. If in doubt it is better to avoid using it.

Flip charts

Flip charts are a similar medium to chalk boards in that they can be used to place emphasis on specific points when presenting information. The charts can be prepared in advance if there are key areas that will be usefully highlighted on one large page. This medium is particularly useful for the speaker leading a session in which audience participation is required and they wish to note down ideas generated for future discussion. This approach may be well suited to a small discussion group.

Overhead projector (OHP)

The overhead projector (OHP) is a popular visual aid in classroom settings and lecture theatres. Consequently this is a useful tool for larger audiences, as the size of the projection on a screen (or plain wall) can be adjusted to meet the size of the room in which the machine is located. In addition, as the speaker does not need to turn away from the audience to use the OHP they can concentrate on audience response more than is possible with a chalk board.

The OHP has other advantages. Although it can be used in the same way as the chalk board for noting key points, acetates for use can be prepared well in advance of the lecture. Prepared acetates can serve to give an instant *aide mémoire* if the headings are related closely to the content of the lecture. It has also been noted that a picture is worth a thousand words. A clear concise diagram can have a much stronger impact on the audience than a long, detailed explanation. Consequently this is particularly useful to researchers looking for ways to summarise findings.

A major disadvantage of using the overhead projector is that, as with all mechanical objects, it may break down at a crucial moment. If the speaker is not skilled in maintaining this equipment, and carrying out procedures such as changing light bulbs, it is useful to check if there will be a technician available to help and advise. To be prepared, if a lecturer is planning to use this tool, it is always as well for them to think in advance how they will present the lecture in case the equipment fails.

The second potential disadvantage of using an OHP relates to the preparation of the acetates. There are many complex techniques that can be used but to enhance the quality of acetates prepared by hand it will be useful to consider a few simple points:

1.   Do not attempt to put too much information on the acetate. The impact of a few key words is stronger than a sheet filled with detailed information.

2.   The size of the letters/figures used is important. If very small writing is used it may not be seen at the back of the room. There are no rigid rules to follow, but letters should be at least 5 mm in size and it is better to print than to link letters. A variety of lettering sets available on the market can be useful

if looking for a 'professional' finish to acetates, and can be particularly so if the lecturer's own writing is not adequate. It is advisable to test your acetates for clarity on an OHP well before the lecture to allow time for improvement if necessary.

3.   There are a variety of pens available for preparing acetates. Spirit-based pens tend to give a sharper finish but are not as easy to clean if a mistake is made. Water-based pens are easy to use but can be easily smudged if the acetate gets damp. The choice of pens may be affected by what is available at the time of preparation.

4.   Pens come in a variety of colours and it is tempting to use several colours when preparing acetates. For impact, however, it is better to use a limited range of only two or three colours, as this is less distracting for the audience. Also, there is a need to take care in the choice of colours used. Some, such as yellow, may seem appealing when preparing acetates but they do not show up well on the screen. Light colours may be better used for shading words or pictures to create visual impact.

5.   Diagrams and pictures can be demonstrated well with acetates as long as they too are kept simple. If demonstrating research results, graphs or histograms can be transferred onto an acetate to provide a clear source of reference for the audience. More than one acetate can be used to 'build up' a picture by placing a second on top of the first. Although a useful technique it is important not to overdo this. Too many acetates may serve to confuse if the detail becomes too complex. Also, the finished product may not be clear as the light source will become diluted by the thickness of the acetates.

6.   Cartoons are a useful way of giving impact to a message, or simply to introduce some variety into a presentation. These are easily traced from original pictures if using acetates. However, cartoons should be used sparingly. While the occasional picture can have a big impact, too many can be tedious for the audience and distract from the main theme of the presentation.

7.   Finally, there are some general points in relation to using an OHP that should be briefly outlined. First, practice using the OHP before an important lecture. It can be irritating to an audience if the speaker is fumbling around trying to get the machine to work. Secondly, speakers should be prepared to raise their voice if the OHP has a noisy fan system, as some of the older models have.

It is important that the lecturer does not stand in front of the OHP when giving a presentation. If they do, all the hard work of preparation will be in vain for the audience will only see the outline of the speaker's body. Equally, it is important not to cover the acetate with a hand when displaying information on the OHP. First, because it is distracting and secondly, if the speaker is very nervous when talking their shaking hand will be well magnified for all to see; it is far better to use a small object such as a pencil to emphasise a word on your acetate. If this is done the lecturer can rest their hand on the side of the machine, an approach that can help to reduce tremor.

Gradual exposure of information on an OHP is a useful way of focusing audience attention. This is easily done by covering the key point with paper and uncovering the words one at a time.

Finally, avoid looking into the light of the OHP as this can be blinding to the speaker and take concentration away from the audience. Practising beforehand allows the speaker to check these points and also gives an opportunity to see if acetates are clear and easy to read when positioned on the OHP. Familiarity with working with prepared acetates will help to increase confidence when giving a lecture.

Slides

In a large audience the use of slides offers an effective means of ensuring that everyone can see information. If slides are to be used it is important that this is considered well in advance, because they take some time to prepare. As with acetates the amount of information on a slide should be kept to a minimum, although it is possible to use complex tables for reference purposes. When presenting research findings issues related to presentation of tables and graphs in Chapter 8 should be considered, for the same principles apply when using slides. Slides can be used for written statements and for pictorial demonstration. If, for any reason, pictures of individuals are to be included in a presentation speakers should ensure that specific permission to use that material has been given and that, where necessary, confidentiality is maintained. For example, if a nurse has undertaken a study into a new treatment for pressure sores she may want to show a picture of a patient before and after that treatment. She would need to obtain that patient's permission to exhibit the picture and may need to deface it to protect the patient's identity.

There is, of course, only value in showing pictures if they demonstrate what you want them to show. Poor quality slides are better not used. The disadvantage in using slides is coping with the technology. It may give the speaker more confidence if they have placed their own slides in the projector, for at least they will then know that they are in the right order and position in the projector. This will also give the opportunity to practice changing slides and adjusting lighting. It is advisable to do this before the presentation.

Hand-outs

Hand-outs which give additional information can be useful to the audience but, as they can be costly, it is important to consider carefully whether the use is appropriate. If hand-outs are used the lecturer should consider carefully when they will be circulated. If they have been designed to save the audience taking notes it is no good circulating them at the end of the lecture after the audience has been busily writing down everything that has been said. Alternatively, if the information on the hand-out is supplementary to the talk then it would be appropriate to circulate this when the lecture is finished. The audience should be told if there is a hand-out available and where and when it will be circulated.

Poster displays

It is common practice in conferences for room to be set aside for poster displays. A poster display is not an aid to help in presentation of a lecture; rather, it is an alternative medium by which research findings, or a specific area of development in nursing, can be shared with colleagues. Presentation in this way incorporates both written and presentation skills. The emphasis is on the posters which should convey the information in a clear and unambiguous way. If summarising a research project for a poster display then the same guidelines as those given for writing a research report apply. Key points should be specifically highlighted to give instant visual impact to the reader and, in relation to this, other information should be kept to a minimum. The idea is to give a concise overview of the subject in such a way that it is appealing to the eye. Supplementary material can be made available in the form of hand-outs if necessary. If a researcher was asked to do a poster display of their work then the organiser would assume that they would be available to talk to people interested in the study and results. So, although this method of presentation may not be as threatening as giving a lecture, it still requires an ability to communicate well.

The audio-visual aids discussed above are the most commonly used equipment by lecturers. The issues raised in relation to using these are of necessity limited in their scope; their use and abuse is a subject worthy of much more detailed exploration but space has allowed only an overview in this text. Confidence with this equipment only comes with practice and the skills of presenting information can be developed with experience. There are people who will be able to help and advise about preparing material for presentation in lectures, be that in a medical illustration department in a hospital, an audio-visual technician in a school of nursing, a teacher or simply a colleague who has had some experience of lecturing. If a nurse in a position to share knowledge with colleagues makes use of these resources they will find that they help to facilitate a good quality presentation.

Summary

This chapter has explored the presentation skills required by nurses who are in a position to share knowledge with their colleagues. Exploration of writing skills are extended beyond that of research for it is felt that if a nurse is not skilled at writing in general she may have difficulty in writing for research. Specific areas of writing for research discussed in this chapter have included the literature review, research proposal and research reports. Skills of verbal presentation have included an overview of lecture preparation and presentation. The use of audio-visual aids to facilitate the quality of presentation has been outlined. Although by no means a definitive outline on the subject some key areas have been explored and useful tips given.

Further reading

Clancy, J. and Ballard, B. (1983) *How to Write Essays: A practical guide for students*, Longman Cheshire, Melbourne.
Cormak, D.F.S. (1984) *Writing for Nursing and Allied Professions*, Blackwell Scientific, Oxford.
Gowers, E. (1977) *The Complete Plain Words*, Penguin, Buckinghamshire.
Jay, A. (1985) *Effective Presentation: The communication of ideas by words and visual aids*, BIM (British Institute of Management), London.

10   Change theory and research

The interest in change theory, which has developed over recent years, has led to the recognition that approaches adopted to making changes in practice can play a major part in determining the success, or otherwise, of any change process. It has been suggested by theorists that if a planned approach is taken the chances of successful implementation of that change process are greatly increased.

The purpose of this chapter is to outline some of the key areas that should be considered when planning changes in nursing practice. This is seen as being an important inclusion in a book on research because once the need to change practices as a result of research studies has been identified, the most effective ways of introducing that change should be considered.

The first part of the chapter will address the subject of change theory while subsequent sections will consider the application of this theory to effecting changes in nursing practice. Examples related to research will be used as appropriate throughout the text.

What is change?

Change is an alteration in the pattern of events in a given situation. It is ever-present and, as part of the normal pattern of life, can be seen as sequential or developmental. In experiencing changes in life events of today are directly affected by our experiences of yesterday. Consequently, we are not generally aware of the changes around us that develop slowly on a day-to-day basis. There are, however, times when we will be aware of changes. This is when situations occur in which change is dramatically imposed upon us at an individual level. For example, we hear of cases in which people become rich overnight and subsequently radically changed their life-style. On a less pleasant note there are unfortunate victims of circumstances whose lives change radically as a result of an accident to themselves or someone near to them. The person who becomes severely disabled as a result of a road traffic accident, for example, will face a very different world to the one in which they previously had control over all aspects of everyday life.

Although these examples are extreme they serve to illustrate why we need to have a knowledge of change theory. We are all faced with developmental changes and, equally, there are times in life when we have all had to face more radical changes. The ways in which we have coped with these situations depend largely on our own coping mechanisms. It is because of individual variations in response to change that study of change theory is now seen to be important to nurses. When working with people we need to understand those mechanisms that enable individuals to react positively or negatively to change in their lives.

Change and the individual

One way in which psychologists explain how people react to change is by analysing attitudes and behaviour. The way in which people behave is generally seen as a good indicator of their attitudes. It is expected that if an individual holds a particular belief then their behaviour would be consistent with that belief. However, this is not always the case and it is not uncommon for people to have strong beliefs or attitudes about something yet act in a manner that is inconsistent with this. For example, a nurse may indicate in group discussion that she believes most strongly in encouraging independence in the patients in her ward. When observed, however, this same nurse may be seen to be dressing the patient rather than allowing individual patients to dress themselves. The nurse may be able to give a rational reason for this apparent inconsistency in stated beliefs and actual behaviour. She may state, for example, that there were not enough nurses on the ward on this one occasion to allow the patient to dress himself for this takes more time to supervise than to do; this serves to indicate how a strongly stated attitude may fail to be demonstrated in practice.

It is important that the nurse is aware of inconsistencies in human nature when planning to implement changes in practice. Issues related to this will be discussed further in the section on implementing change.

Change and the organisation

The study of change in organisations has provided a focus for management theorists for some time, for it is felt that a good understanding of how change occurs can be of benefit when making future plans for the development of the organisation. As the National Health Service consists of many organisations such as hospitals, studies of change theory are pertinent to such environments.

At both an individual and an organisational level the principles of change can be seen to have similar application and effect. As with the individual, changes within an organisation can be developmental: as time passes new approaches to work evolve. However, organisations can also be faced with a more dramatic change process as the result of external factors. It may be suggested that it is the more dramatic type of change that forms the base for change theory and gives the focus for studies of planned change within organisations. It is to be expected that if there is potential for inconsistency at an individual level then the same problem can be applied at an organisational level, for organisations are made up of collections of individuals.

Theorists have attempted to categorise changes in organisations and it will be useful to review these categories in more detail. For the most part in life individuals seek to maintain a balance, or status quo. This serves to give us a stable base from which to organise our lives and to view the world. The same is true of organisations. There is a normal balance of factors affecting the way in which an organisation works; all these contribute towards maintaining the status quo. If a change of routine is introduced into that organisation then sections of it would strive to seek a new balance. For example, the introduction of a new treatment may generate conflict within the hospital because it may mean that previously used methods are no longer used. Consequently resulting instability may lead to conflicts as staff work to achieve a new status quo. It is as a result of conflict generated because of changes within organisations that leads some theorists to suggest that the response to change is a form of conflict resolution as that organisation seeks to find a new balance. Nurses faced with changing practice as a result of new knowledge of research may experience this conflict within themselves and their colleagues as they attempt to change traditional practices.

An alterantive way in which change can be viewed at an organisational level is to use systems theory. Although this can be a complex approach to understand, if studied in depth it provides a useful means of analysing organisational change. The basic idea of systems theory is that many parts contribute towards the whole. Thus, in a health care setting many wards, units, laboratories and departments contribute towards making this functional system known as a hospital. Changes in one part of the system will have an impact on the remaining parts. For example, recent technological advances have allowed techniques to be developed that monitor cerebral structure without the use of invasive techniques. The result of these scanning facilities in many hospitals is that, whereas people were once admitted to hospital to undergo potentially dangerous investigations, the tests can be performed painlessly on an out-patient basis. Therefore, changes that have occurred within the 'system' include a reduction in the number of patients admitted to hospital for invasive exploration of cerebral structure. This in turn has an impact on all other departments providing facilities within the hospital. In the out-patient department, for example, there is a change in the number and type of patients undergoing investigation. This may lead to the need to employ extra personnel in that department to care for the people undergoing such investigations.

The study of change in organisations has indicated that if all relevant factors are considered before the changes occur the outcomes are more likely to be positive. In other words, unplanned change can be more difficult to cope with than planned change. Strategies that can be used to introduce changes in practice can be of benefit to the nurse researcher faced with the problem of changing practice to meet present-day knowledge.

Using change theory

It may be useful to take this review of change one step further and consider the benefits of planned change in the health care setting and to identify how theories of change can help the nurse to utilise research findings in her work.

In general, it is assumed that the purpose of planned change is to improve a situation for the better. Planned change is a deliberate act in which the stages of the change process have been well thought out and appropriate strategy plans for action made. This process is consultative and thus all parties involved in the change process are also involved in the action plan. It is worth considering this further in relation to individual experiences. At some time in their career, most nurses will have worked in an environment in which decisions were made without consultation with them. For example, plans to change the method of organising work in a ward or unit may have been introduced without consultation between the ward sister and the staff. The result of this situation may be that staff follow new ideas when the ward sister is on duty, but return to the old ways in her absence.

This same pattern would no doubt show itself if one member of a ward or unit team decided to implement some aspect of research in nursing practice without proper communication among the team. Obviously, this would do little to promote research awareness and utilisation in the group of nurses concerned. Factors related to planning change will be discussed below but first it is worth considering briefly the roles that may be adopted by nurses involved in change.

The role of the nurse in implementing change

Any nurse may be involved in the change process but the role will differ depending on whether the nurse is initiating, or simply participating in, the change process. There are several titles commonly used in describing roles in change. The title of 'change agent' is used to indicate that a member of an organisation has a specific responsibility for change. This may be seen as a formal role in which the person has been employed specifically for the purpose of initiating change. Alternatively, a nurse who has a progressive outlook in her work and is constantly alert to developing new initiatives in practice may be seen as a change agent in the informal sense. She has not been employed specifically as a change agent but her professional awareness and motivation is such that she initiates change, in practice, as part of normal routine.

The role of the nurse participating in change can be further analysed to identify other characteristics. The result of such an analysis by Ottoway (1980) identifies three groups: change generators, change implementers and change adopters. Change generators identifies the group of people who have the ideas. A research nurse working on a specific project may fall into this category. For example, the early research work undertaken by Norton *et al.* (1975) into pressure area care can be seen to have generated much awareness in nursing practice into this aspect of care. Although considerable work into this subject has been undertaken it can subsequently be seen that in this instance Norton may be seen as the generator of these ideas.

The nurse who takes ideas for practice and plans to use them within the unit can be described as a change implementer. In some units nurses are employed specifically for this purpose. The nurse who uses the research into pressure area care to help to plan a strategy for improved care within a unit may be seen to fulfil this role. Change adopters perhaps represent the majority of practising nurses who are exposed to change. They themselves may not have generated ideas for change and may not have been responsible for organising the implementation of change but they are actively involved in carrying out any changes in practice in their own clinical area. Some texts on change theory describe this role as one supporting change and thus use the title 'change supporter'.

Although the differing titles noted above are useful when analysing the role of the nurse in implementing change, when discussing the change process in this text the title 'change agent' will be used to describe the nurse who is initiating changes in practice. It is acknowledged that the change agent could be both a change generator and a change implementer. The change agent may be someone employed within the organisation, such as a ward sister or a nursing officer, or someone brought in by management to act in a consultative capacity to guide a change in practice.

Characteristics of a change agent

At whatever level the change agent functions within the nursing hierarchy there are some common characteristics that she should have. The first characteristic required in a change agent is an enormous amount of energy, for this is an essential component to any change strategy. This should be coupled with enthusiasm, which is essential to sustain energy when in the midst of a change process. It is most important that the change agent has credibility in the eyes of those people with whom they are working. If changing practice in nursing as a result of research the change agent would require credibility as a nurse, but in addition it may be expected that they have a good working knowledge of research-based practices. Credibility does not necessarily mean that the nurse is a subject specialist, rather it may imply that she is able to use, identify and utilise expert help when necessary. As communication and education is also a crucial part of the change process then the change agent must also possess good interpersonal skills.

Change theories

The subject of change has proved a fascination for theorists for some years and there are many texts available which outline some of the seminal work in this field. As this is a useful formula there is no apology for lack of original thought in following the same sequence in this book by outlining change theories before application to practice is considered. The classic work on change theory is credited to Lewin (1951). His analysis of change offers a very simple model for practitioners. Lewin describes three stages to the change process to which the analogy of a melting ice cube is applied.

In the first stage the need for change is identified and the process begins. In relating this to Lewin's work there is a challenge to the accepted order of things with the result that the identifiable routine begins to change. In other words, the 'ice-cube' begins to melt. Prior to the implementation of change there is an assumed stability in an environment – a familiar pattern of work in which the norms and patterns of behaviour are firmly established. The challenge to the accepted order can cause disruption in the environment and consequently a good deal of sensitivity is needed on the part of the change agent at this stage, as it is sometimes threatening to upset the status quo.

In the second stage the 'ice cube' melts further. The norms within the working situation are slowly beginning to change. As the change strategy is introduced those people within the situation may be experiencing uncertainty and doubts as their normal pattern of life is changing about them. Uncertainty can be anticipated even when there is full group commitment to the change process.

In the third stage a new stability has been established. The change strategy has been implemented and a new pattern of 'norms' emerges. The process of change has resulted in a different routine or approach which is clearly distinguished from the previous pattern of organisation. The ice cube has assumed a different shape.

Planning for change will be discussed below, but first it might be useful to give an example to illustrate how Lewin's theory of change can be applied to an attempt to change one area of practice in nursing.

It is now fairly common practice in many nursing units to undertake audits to monitor the quality of care provided. The research tool used for this purpose may vary but most of these will incorporate a review of the knowledge base of practice. Following a clinical audit it may be noted on one unit, Ward X, that the approach to nursing practice is based on traditional patterns of organising work simply because it 'has always been done that way'. A new manager may feel that this approach is no longer consistent with present-day expectations of care and that something must be done to increase research awareness among the staff. Her goal might be to introduce practices based on research knowledge rather than the rituals and routines that have been the norm. Consequently, the manager may develop a planned change strategy, and may also plan to act as a change agent to implement this change. The process of 'unfreezing' has begun.

The process of planned change is deliberate, collaborative and works towards improvement. There are many aspects that would need to be considered and it is essential that all those involved in the change process are consulted at every stage as a strategy is devised and implemented. The manager would, therefore, discuss all relevant issues and ideas with staff, invite participation and ensure that they are all involved in every stage of development.

As the change strategy is implemented the unit will be moving from the old to the new order of practice. Conflicts may arise during this transition as staff work towards a new 'balance' in their approach to work. It would be recognised that individual security could be upset by changes in the environment and so the role of the change agent is crucial in ensuring that staff have the necessary education and information to help them to achieve this change. There is a need to give support to all those involved during a change process.

The final stage of the change process, refreezing, is reached when the new pattern of practice is implemented in the unit. In this example the anticipated result of the planned change would be a more questioning approach to work and practices based on an awareness of research. There would be a new stability in the unit as this method of work becomes the normal approach.

In this example it can be seen that the aim is to change one situation to another in which a different pattern of working emerges. There is a new shape to the 'ice cube' or the routine of practice. Other theorists have developed Lewin's three-stage process further to highlight all the factors that must be considered in relation to planning change. For a more in-depth review of this subject a further reading section is included at the end of the chapter. The remainder of this chapter will consider some aspects that should be considered when planning a change in practice in a unit.

Planning a change strategy

In implementing change the two approaches that can be clearly identified are the 'top down' or a 'bottom up' approach. The former indicates some form of senior managerial input in which change is directed from a position of power within a hierarchical setting. There are situations in which this method of implementing change is necessary. However, to be effective the person responsible must be skilled in ensuring that the change is collaborative and that all those people involved in the planned action have some input into the planning.

The 'bottom up' approach implies that initiatives are taken at 'shop floor' level. It is generally felt that change generated from the bottom up is more likely to succeed than that imposed from the 'top down' by those in a position of power. It is important to note, however, that changes generated from the bottom up are only likely to succeed in the long term if management are supportive to initiatives undertaken. With this knowledge of change theory a manager may introduce ideas to staff in such a way that those most involved in the change process feel they have some control over new initiative.

Determining an action plan for change

One essential aspect to be considered when planning change is how best to use the knowledge available. The nurse wishing to implement changes based on research findings will need to use nursing knowledge, knowledge of research and a knowledge of how to implement change in practice.

The first aspect that must be identified in any change strategy is to identify exactly the problem that demands the intervention of a change strategy. Having done that the next step, as in any problem-solving process, is to identify the goal of any action that is taken. The problem raised in the example of the ward audit used above may have been that there was a lack of research awareness in Ward X. Having determined the problem area the nurse manager determined her goal. This was to create an environment in which research awareness and knowledge-based practice was evident in the care given in the ward.

To achieve the goal the change agent would need to review many aspects relating to both the organisation and individuals working within it. As noted earlier, one view of change adopts a systems approach in which the impact of change in one area can have an impact on many other parts of the organisation. Consequently the nurse change agent must consider this. If she is to encourage research-based practice in one unit, she needs to consider the effect of this in other areas. For example, if she wishes to increase the knowledge of her staff she may want to send them on study days to update their knowledge. This will have an effect on the number of staff available as a resource to the hospital. In addition, it may put a demand on teaching staff who may be required to plan and facilitate the study sessions.

The method of administration within the organisation is another crucial factor that must be considered. A rigid, hierarchical management style may not be helpful when attempting to instigate changes in a unit. In contrast an open, democratic management system in which change is encouraged is likely to be supportive of unit-based initiatives.

Management styles within the multi-disciplinary team must also be reviewed. Obviously, if the health care team works well together then changes within one group will be more likely to be accepted by the other members of the team. If one group dominates the team this may be detrimental to other team members. The needs of all team members should be considered in a planned change programme. The number of people who are to be involved in a change process will also play a part in determining the success or otherwise of planned change strategies. A community nurse working with a small group of colleagues in a discreet geographical area may find it easier to work at effecting change with her small number of colleagues than would a sister working in an intensive care unit employing sixty members of staff.

The timing of any planned change strategy is also crucial. For example, staff are not likely to respond well to a proposed meeting to discuss plans for change at a time of extremely high work-load and staff shortages. It is possible that excuses are constantly made as to why a given time is not suitable for change strategies to be implemented, but the skilled change agent will recognise any such delaying tactics.

It is expected that the change agent will review the proposals for change from every angle. In so doing any precedents set in this area would be considered. It is useful in any planned change to be able to share in the successes or otherwise of those people who have undergone similar experiences. Sharing at this stage can help to avoid repetition of mistakes. It can also help to avoid any pitfalls that have been identified by others who have had similar experiences. The costs of any initiatives should also be considered in depth. For example, there may be implications in preparing the staff for change that will incur costs in sending them on courses to update their knowledge.

The change agent must be realistic in terms of what is achievable with a planned strategy. It would be totally unrealistic to anticipate changing a ward area in which there was very little awareness of nursing research to one in which practices reflect an approach produced by nurses with a long experience in research-based practices in a three-month period. The aims of the planned change should clearly reflect realistic, achievable goals.

The change agent should determine individual talents and abilities in the group involved in the change process so that these may be utilised in any subsequent action plan. Some understanding of psychology of both individuals and groups can be usefully deployed at this stage. Individual attitudes play a large part in determining the success of any change venture and it may be necessary for the change agent to plan means of overcoming any resistance to change. Some nurses may be resistant to research-based practice for, as discussed in Chapter 2, they may simply not have the knowledge base and thus see research as something distant from their everyday work. Others may be resistant to change simply because they are afraid of what the implications mean for them and how, for example, their role will be affected. Change will result in uncertainly simply because it upsets the status quo and changes normal, comfortable routines for those involved. This means that all those involved in change, even if they are simply involved in adopting change, will need energy to cope with the altered pattern of their lives.

Group dynamics also play a part in determining the success of planned change. It is well documented that people may behave differently in groups to the way in which they behave as individuals. Consequently, it is important to analyse the working group situation. If the more vocal members of a group are resistant to change they may influence the views of their colleagues in the group. This reinforces the point made earlier in that another skill required by a change agent is the ability to communicate well at individual and group levels; indeed, not simply to communicate but to be able to use a full range of diplomatic skills when leading a group through a change process.

Having completed a thorough analysis of the situation the change agent should be able to list all the constraining forces opposing the success of the change and all the resources that might facilitate the success of the plan. It may be suggested that if the resources exceed the constraining forces the chances of success are increased. However, this is not always so and consequently each

Constraining forces	Resources
Rigid ward routine	Enthusiastic Sister
Poor knowledge of research	Post basic students
Staff in post for many years	District research nurse
Medical staff traditional in approach	Funding available to support staff education
Very busy workload	Supportive management

Figure 10.1 Introducing research-based practice to Ward X

case must be judged on individual merits. It is useful to list these opposing forces alongside each other. An example of this is shown in Figure 10.1, which illustrates the factors identified by the nurse planning to increase the research awareness within her unit.

In determining what is possible the change agent will make any modifications to her plan at the outset. In addition, the change agent will consider what aspects of the plan are essential and what could be modified in the light of discussion and planning with all those involved in the changes. This will allow some alterations to be made if the rest of the staff involved in the change process are not totally in support of the planned change.

Implementing change

As with all problem-solving processes the quality of the preparation will have a direct impact on the outcome of the planned change. The planning stage is crucial and should not be underestimated by nurses responsible for implementing change in nursing practices.

Communication and education are crucial factors that should be continued throughout the change process. The way in which these aspects are handled will make the difference between success or failure of the venture. It cannot be stressed often enough that all staff involved in the change process must be consulted at every stage and, wherever possible, their ideas noted and utilised in the process. Co-operation is greatly increased if people feel that they are working with ideas generated from them.

It should also be noted that throughout the implementation process the change agent must be available to give support to those involved as they face the uncertainties engendered by changes in their environment.

Finally, it is essential that the change agent is able to recognise those factors that contribute towards resistance to the planned change. Recognition of these in the early stages can do much to help to avoid the problems that can occur once resistance becomes firmly established.

Resistance to change

Knowledge of those factors that may cause resistance to change is essential to any person wishing to develop a change strategy. This knowledge allows the change agent to make appropriate plans to meet with resistance should it occur, for if resistance is present and not detected early enough the result will be great difficulty in implementing change. In their outline of resistance to change Lancaster and Lancaster (1982) highlight the fact that not all resistance is bad in that it identifies a need to keep a close assessment on the ideas for change and for those initiating changes to be prepared to support their ideas as necessary.

Opposing and supporting factors that should be considered before embarking on a change programme can be analysed carefully to anticipate any factor that might result in resistance to the planned change.

Several factors are seen to relate to resistance. The first of these is perhaps the degree of change planned. For example, a nurse manager may want to change the pattern of shifts worked within a unit by ten minutes at each end of the day. This change will have implications for staff and consequently may result in much debate and discussion. Subsequently this change may be easily adopted, for it does not represent a major change of routine for those staff concerned. However, a proposal to change working hours to fit the continental pattern in which nurses work one of three shifts over the 24-hour period may have a greater impact on those nurses concerned, for it may represent a need to completely change their daily routine. Of the two situations outlined above the latter example is more likely to generate resistance for it represents the greater change and therefore is more likely to be disruptive for those staff concerned. If the proposed change is seen as likely to have an effect on individual freedom and cause inconvenience to the individual it is more likely to result in resistance.

Previous experience will have an effect on the way in which people respond to change. It is not uncommon for people to take a rather negative stance to proposed change, taking the view that they have 'seen it all before' and therefore the outcome is anticipated. This negative stance is more likely to occur if the individual experience of change has not been positive in the past.

There are several other reasons why resistance to change might develop. Fear is frequently cited as one of these. Uncertainty results in fear, for the outcome is unknown. This is especially so if the status quo is threatened and, as noted earlier, individuals are not sure what the change will mean to them. Another factor is lack of knowledge. This may be related to knowledge of the subject area of the change, or, more simply, lack of knowledge relating to the purpose of the change. The lack of clearly defined goals in the change programme can have a negative impact. The example of changing shift patterns noted above illustrates this point. If the recipients of the change plan are only told that there is to be a change in the duty shifts then they are likely to expect the most complex of the choices and may be resisting the change before they are fully aware of the proposed plans.

The role of the change agent is another aspect to consider. Mauksch and Miller (1981) note that it is not uncommon for a change agent to be searching for a rational explanation as to why a change strategy has failed, drawing on their knowledge of the points noted above. What may not be obvious to the change agent is that the failure lies in themselves, for they do not have the necessary skill or have not deployed the appropriate strategy to implement their programme of change.

Types of resistance to change

Resistance to change can be seen either in the way that groups function or in the behaviour of individuals within groups. For the purpose of explanation resistance to change can be divided into two categories, active or passive resistance.

Active resistance means that there is evidence of an individual or a group actively working against the proposed change. This may be seen in the form of disruptive behaviour in which there are obvious attempts to undermine the success of the change. Individuals may become aggressive in their approach to the change agent or, indeed, to those around them who may be seen to be participating in the change.

Passive resistance may be less obvious to the observer. The individual may pay lip service to the change, praising the benefits on one occasion but stating quite different views when out of earshot of the supporters of change. In addition, this individual may not attempt to change their own practice in any way. Apathy or seeming exhaustion may be an indicator of this problem.

Whichever way individuals or groups demonstrate a resistance to change the outcome will be the same: lack of continuity in the change programme, an aspect that is hardly likely to enhance its success.

Maintaining change

One final aspect should be considered in relation to implementing change in practice; that is, maintaining the change once it has been introduced. If the change strategy has been well prepared then the chances of maintaining the change are much increased.

If the change strategy has relied heavily on the commitment and enthusiasm of one person there is a risk that the old order of work may be re-introduced over a period of time. In the example given in this text it is feasible that the research-based practices introduced into one unit may continue as long as the nurse manager holds her post. Unless she has followed a very careful strategy plan to the level at which staff are also committed to the changes the new order of work may not be maintained in her absence.

It is important to maintain constant vigilance until the change strategy has been adopted as the new norm. Positive reinforcement, in which credit is given for efforts made and results noted, is another way of helping to sustain a change in practice. This is useful to those who have experienced personal doubts as a result of the change process.

Change theory and research

It was noted earlier in this book that there are many areas of nursing in which research is seen as a relatively new phenomenon. An increased awareness of research will involve challenging the routines and rituals of practices in nursing (see Chapter 2). It is because of this situation that all the factors outlined above in relation to change theory should be considered carefully by the nurse who wishes to introduce research-based practices to her unit. Individual knowledge of research in a nurse is now an essential prerequisite to practice. However, if that nurse is using an approach reflecting research awareness in isolation then the ultimate impact of her knowledge may be limited for the patients in her care. It is important that all of those nurses caring for the patient take a similar approach to the care given. The information included in this chapter can be applied to any change process within the working environment, but readers are advised to consider carefully the issues raised when considering the use of research in nursing practice. Nurses who are seeking to change practices as a result of their increased knowledge of research should take particular note of the issues discussed.

Summary

This chapter has explored the subject of change theory. There has been an attempt to define change before considering how to use change theory in practice. Aspects to consider in planning a change strategy have been outlined as a guide. Finally it was acknowledged that, although the principles of change are applicable across a wide range of situations, there is a particular need to consider change theory when applying research to nursing practice to ensure consistency in care given.

Further reading

CURN Project (1983) *Using Research to Improve Nursing Practice: a Guide*, Grune & Stratton, Orlando.

Lancaster, J. and Lancaster, W. (eds) (1982) *Concepts for Advanced Nursing Practice. The Nurse as a Change Agent*, C.V. Mosby, St. Louis.

Lewin, K. (1951) *Field Theory in Social Science*, Harper & Row, New York.

Mauksch, I.G. and Miller, M.H. (1981) *Implementing Change in Nursing*, C.V. Mosby, St. Louis.

Norton, D., McLaren, R. and Exton-Smith, A.N. (1975) *An Investigation of Geriatric Nursing Problems in Hospital*, Churchill Livingstone, Edinburgh.

Ottoway, R.N. (1980) *Defining the Change Agent*, Unpublished Research Paper, University of Manchester Institute of Technology, Department of Management Sciences, Manchester.

Index

abstracting services, journals, 59–60
action research, 77–8
Activities of Living (ALs), 22, 23 (Table), 24–6
analysing research data, 94–109
anonymity, writing for publication, 119
applying research in practice, 13–14
approaches to research, 70–4
area of study, defining, 28, 36
audio-visual aids, 123, 124–9
  chalk board, 125
  flip charts, 125–6
  hand-outs, 129
  overhead projector, 126–8
  poster displays, 129
  slides, 128

bar graphs, presentation of data, 100 (Figure), 101
bibliography, 54–5, 65
Bibliography of Nursing Literature, 55
bimodal distribution, 107, 108 (Figure)
body language, 89, 124
books
  connecting reference to reference list, 66–7
  sources of information
    bibliography, 54–5
    directories, 55–6
    library catalogue, 54
    sourcebooks, 56
    statistics, 56
British National Bibliography (BNB), 54–5

case study
  data collection, 75–7
    advantages, 75–6
    disadvantages, 76
    techniques, 76–7
chalk board, using, 125
change
  definition, 131

implementing, 141
  maintaining, 143
  planned, 134, 137, 139
  resistance to, 141–2
  types of, 143
  role of nurse in implementing, 134–5
change agent
  characteristics, 135–6
  definition, 134
change strategy
  planning, 138–43
    determining action plan, 138–41
change theory
  change and the individual, 132
  change and the organisation, 132–4
  research, 143–4
  theories, 136–7
closed questions, 85
common sense, 10–11
computer retrieval systems, 61–3, 64 (Table)
conferences, disseminating research findings, 17
confidentiality, 119
copyright, 49–50
  registration of original material, 67
Copyright, Designs and Patents Act 1988, 49
cost of research, 14
cross-sectional study, 74–5
Crown Copyright material, 50
Cumulative Index of Nursing and Allied Health Literature (CINAHL), 58–9
current awareness services, journals, 60–1
Current Literature on Health Services, 61

data analysis, 45
data collection, 45, 71–93
  action research, 77–8
  case study, 75–7
    advantages, 75–6
    disadvantages, 76
    techniques, 76–7